Myriam Krifa
Mohamed Hedi Ben Cheikh

Applications of artificial intelligence in healthcare

Myriam Krifa
Mohamed Hedi Ben Cheikh

Applications of artificial intelligence in healthcare

Impacts and challenges

ScienciaScripts

Imprint

Cover image: www.ingimage.com

This book is a translation from the original published under ISBN 978-620-2-28258-1.

Publisher:
Sciencia Scripts
is a trademark of
Dodo Books Indian Ocean Ltd. and OmniScriptum S.R.L publishing group

120 High Road, East Finchley, London, N2 9ED, United Kingdom
Str. Armeneasca 28/1, office 1, Chisinau MD-2012, Republic of Moldova, Europe
Managing Directors: Ieva Konstantinova, Victoria Ursu
info@omniscriptum.com

Printed at: see last page
ISBN: 978-620-8-39637-4

CONTENTS

INTRODUCTION

Artificial intelligence is a major revolution today, opening up unprecedented possibilities in the healthcare sector.In this era of increasing digitalisation, its application has become ubiquitous, transforming the way diseases are diagnosed, treated and prevented. In fact, the World Health Organisation (WHO) has already included the development of digital technologies in its 2021-2030 global action plan, underlining their crucial importance in improving the quality of care and patient safety **[1]**.

In addition, the use of machine learning and Big Data analysis in the medical and pharmaceutical fields has opened up a vast field of opportunities. Artificial intelligence (AI) has made it possible not only to automate the search for new drugs, but also to predict and evaluate their efficacy and safety. Similarly, machine learning has made it easier to analyse clinical data, personalise therapies and identify potential interactions between drugs, while Big Data analysis in pharmacovigilance has helped to detect safety problems early on.

At the same time, this technological advance also raises essential questions about regulatory and ethical issues, as well as the limits of its application, particularly in the field of health.

In this work, we explored in depth the theoretical foundations of AI, in particular the Python programming language, machine learning and deep learning. These concepts are essential for understanding the underlying mechanisms of AI and the opportunities for applying them in the medical context. The main objective of this work was to carry out a literature review to describe the most innovative applications of AI and their implications for medical and pharmaceutical practices, while taking a close look at the challenges and issues associated with its use.

1. LANGUAGE PYTHON

1.1.Presentation

Python is a high-level interactive programming language that was created by Guido Van Rossum in 1985 and first published in 1991 as Python 0.9.0 **[2]**. It is dynamically typed, meaning that the user does not need to specify the data type for values stored in the program. Python 2.0 was released in 2000, followed by the 3ème version in 2008, which is not fully compatible with previous versions **[3]**. Python's source code is available under the Python Software Foundation License. It is open source and completely free, even for commercial use, as are its many key scientific libraries. Due to its ease of use, readability and availability on several platforms (Windows, Mac OS, Linux, etc.), Python is widely used in the healthcare field for a variety of applications, including data analysis, statistical modelling and bioinformatics **[4]**.

In 2022, an online repository that stores and hosts Python libraries, called the Python Package Index, reported that Python ranked as the most in-demand programming language **[3]**. This finding is reinforced by the considerable number of jobs reserved for experienced Python developers, exceeding 40,000 positions in the countries surveyed **[3]**. These figures bear witness to the significant impact of this programme in today's landscape, underlining its relevance and the diversity of its applications, particularly in the healthcare sector.

1.2.Basic concepts

A computer language is a system of communication between humans and computers, transforming algorithms into instructions that the computer can use. understand and execute. Unlike natural languages, these instructions must follow strict and precise syntax rules in order to be interpreted correctly by the machine **[5]**. These rules are as follows:

- **End of Lines :** Unlike many other classical languages, Python does not need a semicolon to mark the end of a command line. A simple newline tells the interpreter that the command is finished **[6]**.
- **Indentation**: In the context of programming, indentation refers to the use of white space at the beginning of a line of code to delimit the scope or hierarchical level of the code. It is essential for determining the structure and readability of a program, particularly in languages that rely on it to define the scope of blocks of code, such as Python (**Figure 1**). In most other languages, {} braces are used to

define the scope of a block of code. But in Python, indentation replaces these braces, which makes the code more readable and uncluttered, but also requires careful attention to the consistency of indentation throughout the code **[5]**.

- **Comments:** Any line beginning with a hash '#' in Python is treated as a comment and will be ignored by the interpreter **[6]**.
- **Variables:** In Python, a variable is used to store information, such as a number or a character string. It is declared simply by using the equal sign '=' **[6]**.
- **Data types :** Each variable in Python is associated with a type. Common types include strings, integers, booleans and lists. For example, a Boolean variable can only be "True" or "False", an integer represents numbers without decimal places, and a string can contain text or symbols **[6]**.
- **Operators:** Python uses operators to perform mathematical operations and comparisons. These symbols, such as + ; - ; * ; / ; == or
!=" can be used to manipulate or compare values and variables **[6]**.

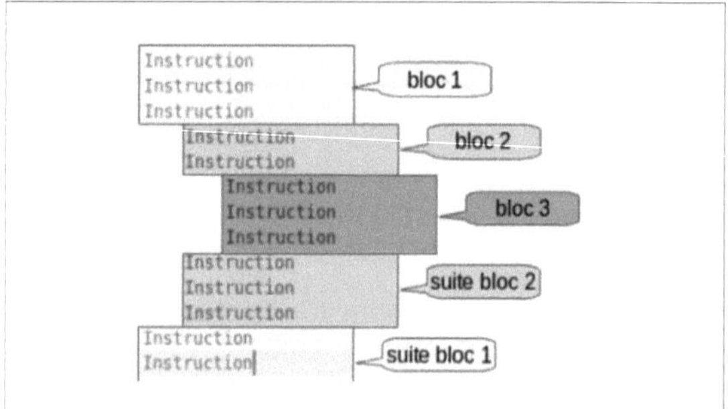

Figure 1: Explanatory example of indentation in computer language [5].

1.3. Libraries

The availability of a variety of libraries specialising in machine learning and other areas of computer science has greatly simplified the development process in Python. These libraries contain ready-to-use functionality such as machine learning algorithms, data visualisation tools, file manipulation functions and much more **[3]**. Because they are available, programmers can avoid having to create functionality from scratch, which considerably reduces the time and effort needed to develop complex new applications. In the field of machine learning, libraries such as TensorFlow, scikit-learn and PyTorch offer ready-to-use implementations of algorithms and data processing techniques **[3]**.

They also provide user-friendly interfaces and advanced features that enable developers to quickly create high-performance machine learning models.

Thanks to this wealth of available resources, Python has become a popular choice for developing machine learning applications. Users can take advantage of these libraries to explore new ideas, quickly experiment with different models, and deploy machine learning solutions in a variety of fields, including healthcare, where Python is increasingly used for tasks such as analysing medical data, predicting disease, and creating diagnostic support systems **[3]**.

1.4. Advantages and disadvantages

1.4.1. Points

Compared with other languages, Python has a number of advantages, not least its variety of available libraries, which have not only reduced the code to a third for the programmer, but also enabled it to achieve the highest level of machine learning **[7]**. In addition, the language frequently uses English-language keywords, which reduces the need for syntactic constructions compared with other languages **[2]**. Python is also interpreted, which means that it is processed at runtime by the interpreter, avoiding the need to compile the program before executing it **[2]**. In other words, with Python there is no need to transform the code into machine language before executing it. The Python interpreter takes care of translating and executing the code directly, which saves time and simplifies the development process. The Python program is also interactive, meaning that users can see the results instantly as they type their code **[2]**.
This makes writing programmes faster and easier, as programmers can quickly test small parts of the code without having to write an entire programme. On the other hand, Python supports the object-oriented programming style, which allows code to be encapsulated within objects that can be manipulated and used in a modular way to solve complex problems **[2]**. Here, the term "object" is a programming paradigm that represents entities that interact with each other and contain both data and functionality. This paradigm makes it possible to model real-world entities in a more natural way.
All these features make Python an ideal language for beginners, as it supports the development of a wide range of applications, from simple word processors to web browsers. It is also highly portable, which means it is compatible with a wide variety of hardware platforms, including Linux, MacOS and Microsoft Windows **[2]**. In addition, it offers a wide range of dynamic data structures such as lists, tuples and dictionaries, which are available as standard and ready to use **[2]**. Finally, Python has many other advantages, including code brevity, support for multiple programming paradigms, a large support community, an extensive third-party library for different areas of work, and dynamic typing that reduces

stress for new programmers by automatically managing data types **[3]**.

1.4.2. Points weaknesses

Despite its many advantages, Python also has a few drawbacks. Firstly, its performance can be inferior to that of compiled languages such as Java, C or C++, due to its interpretation, which can pose challenges for computationally intensive applications such as medical image processing **[3]**.
Furthermore, Python's dynamic typing, while offering greater flexibility in manipulating data types, can also be seen as a drawback in the context of critical software development. for healthcare. This flexibility can lead to errors that are difficult to detect, which can compromise the reliability and security of healthcare applications **[3]**.
Due to its interpreted nature, Python can have limitations when it comes to developing programs that require a graphical user interface. Although libraries such as Tkinter are available to create this type of interface, their performance and fluidity may not be as high as those of compiled languages **[3]**. In addition, the high memory consumption of Python can be a drawback for applications intended to run on mobile devices **[3]**.
Finally, Python does not have as much built-in functionality for accessing and manipulating databases as some other technologies such as Java Database Connectivity and Open Database Connectivity **[3]**. As a result, when developing healthcare applications using Python, manipulators may face additional challenges in effectively integrating databases.
Despite these challenges, Python remains a popular choice for healthcare software development because of its simplicity, flexibility and extensive library of specialist modules.

2. AUTOMATIC LEARNING

2.1. Definition

Machine learning (ML) is an essential branch of artificial intelligence in which computer programs learn from data to perform specific tasks such as classification, prediction or pattern recognition, without being explicitly programmed **[8]**.

This discipline evolved from the first attempts to simulate the human brain using artificial neural networks in the 1950s, to undergo significant expansion from the 2000s onwards, supported by the increase in computing power of computers and the rise of "Big Data" **[8]**.

ML uses mathematical concepts such as statistics, linear algebra and optimisation to create predictive models from the available data. These models are then trained and refined using supervised, unsupervised or reinforcement learning algorithms, depending on the nature of the data and the objectives of the project **[8]**.

In the healthcare sector, ML has many promising applications. For example, it can be used to analyse medical data in order to detect diseases at an early stage, optimise treatments or predict the evolution of certain pathologies in patients. By exploiting large datasets, ML can also contribute to pharmaceutical research by identifying new drugs or speeding up the discovery process for innovative molecules. In this way, it represents a powerful tool for extracting valuable information from complex data to improve decisions, processes and results in a variety of fields, including healthcare.

2.2. Learning model automatic

Machine learning is not limited to a series of algorithms, but rather follows a sequence of methodical steps. According to Isaac Tonyloi **[9]**, a mathematician with expertise in statistics and computer programming, the steps involved in building an ML model are shown in **Figure 2** .

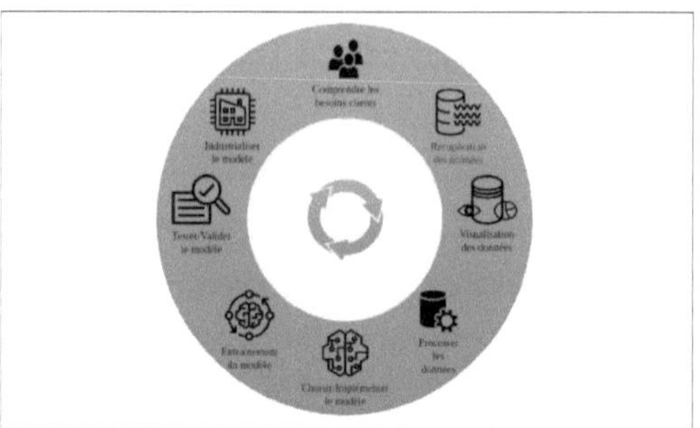

Figure 2: Life cycle of a machine learning model [9].

❖ **Stage 1** involves identifying the problem to be solved and acquiring the data, the quality and quantity of which will influence the success of the project. It is therefore important to collect relevant data while avoiding bias.

❖ **Stage 2** is data analysis and exploration. This phase reveals imbalances in the input or output data, clusters that need to be treated separately, or anomalies that need to be detected.

❖ **Step 3** involves pre-processing and cleaning the data. The data collected requires prior adjustments. This includes removing unnecessary attributes, dealing with missing values, and normalising or standardising the data for consistency. When preparing data for modelling, Python provides libraries and modules that make this process very simple, with Pandas, NumPy and Matplotlib at the top of the list.

❖ **Step 4** involves separating or dividing the data into training data and the test ones. The most commonly used ratio is 80%/20% for the These are the "training set" and "test set" respectively.

❖ **Step 5** coincides with the selection or construction of a learning model appropriate to the problem and the data. Choices may include supervised, unsupervised or reinforcement learning models.

❖ **Step 6** involves training, evaluating and optimising the model. Evaluating the accuracy of the model requires the use of appropriate metrics. If necessary, adjustments must be made to improve the model's performance, and these steps repeated until satisfaction is achieved.

❖ **Step 7** involves testing the model on the dataset to verify its effectiveness and its ability to generate consistent results on a dataset that is unknown to it.

❖ **Step 8** is the deployment of the model in production for predictions, with the possibility of retraining and improvement based on new data.

Although these 8 steps are complex and require expertise, there are tools, such as "Auto ML" or "No Code", that automate model building to make machine learning more accessible. These tools include open source platforms such as PyCaret, Jarvis, pSeven, MLBox, Knime and DataRobot **[10]**.

2.3. Learning algorithms

Once all the data has been collected, various machine learning approaches are used, including three in particular algorithms: supervised, unsupervised and reinforcement learning (**Table I**).

Table I: Comparison between the main machine learning algorithms [11].

	Learning supervised	Learning unsupervised	Learning by reinforcement
Definition	The algorithm	The algorithm is	The algorithm interacts
	learns from	trained from	with its
	of data	data not	environment in
	labelled	labelled without	carrying out actions and
		indications	by learning from its
		specific	mistakes and successes
Types of	Regression and	Association and	Based on a system of
problems	classification	clustering	award
Type of	Input data	Input data	No data
data	labelled	non-labelled	provided in advance
Approach	Study the	Discover the	Learns a strategy
	sub	reasons common to	behaviour in
	that bind	within the data	experience function
	data in	input	and
	entry to labels		rewards received

2.3.1. Supervised learning

In supervised machine learning, the model is trained on labelled data, which means that the input data is associated with pre-existing output labels. The algorithm designer creates a training set from the data of interest. For example, in a binary classification task, the data may be labelled as "True" for positive cases and "False" for negative cases. "False" for negative cases **[12]**. Once the data cleaning and training have been completed, the algorithm is no longer updated, which means there is no more learning. Next, the The accuracy of the model is assessed against a separate data set, called the 'test set', which has not been used during training.

If the accuracy, specificity and sensitivity of the model are deemed sufficient, the algorithm is ready to be implemented in a real environment. If not, the designer needs to review the attributes selected/labelled and may need to re-examine the training process to improve model performance **[12]**.

In the healthcare context, labels are often medical results, diagnoses or predictions about patients. For example, the algorithm can be trained on patient data including characteristics such as age, gender, medical history, etc., as well as labels indicating each patient's diagnosis. Once the algorithm has been trained, it can be used to predict diagnoses for new patients based on their characteristics **[13]**.

It should also be noted that supervised learning can be used for regression tasks in addition to classification tasks. In this case, the model is trained to predict a numerical value rather than assigning class labels. For example, a supervised regression model could be used to predict a hospital patient's length of stay based on their own medical data **[14]**.

In short, supervised learning enables a computer system to learn from labelled data and make predictions or classifications on new data.

2.3.2. Unsupervised learning

Unsupervised learning is a branch of machine learning where computers explore datasets without pre-existing labels to identify intrinsic patterns, hidden structures or meaningful groupings **[11]**. Unlike supervised learning, where In unsupervised learning, the data is unlabelled, unclassified and uncategorized **[11]**. Unsupervised learning methods cannot be directly applied to a regression or classification problem, as the output values are not known. Common algorithms used in unsupervised learning include clustering and association **[11]**.

Clustering can be used to identify natural groups or clusters of similar data within a dataset. Clustering can be used to group genes according to their similar expression profiles **[12]**. This allows researchers to discover new disease subtypes or identify common biological pathways associated with specific medical conditions.

Association, on the other hand, is a technique that aims to discover interesting relationships or correlations between different elements in a data set. Unlike 'clustering', which groups similar data according to their common characteristics, association focuses on identifying specific combinations of elements that occur together in a significant way. In the field of health, this technique can be used to discover links and relationships between different symptoms or risk factors for disease. For example, by analysing patients' computerised medical records, we can use these algorithms to identify combinations of symptoms frequently observed in patients suffering from certain diseases **[13]**.

In summary, unsupervised learning offers a powerful means of exploring and discovering hidden structures or patterns from unlabelled healthcare data, which can provide valuable information for clinical decision-making, medical research and care management **[14]**.

2.3.3. Learning by reinforcement

Reinforcement learning (RL) is a very broad sub-field of machine learning. It is a type of dynamic programming that trains algorithms using a system of rewards and penalties **[15]**. He improves his algorithm over time thanks to a constant feedback loop. Indeed, AR is a computational approach to learning by doing in the absence of a training dataset, i.e. learning by experience, by trial and error, to determine which actions produce the greatest reward. AR is made up of several interacting components resulting in a dynamic learning process (**Figure 3**) **[16]**.

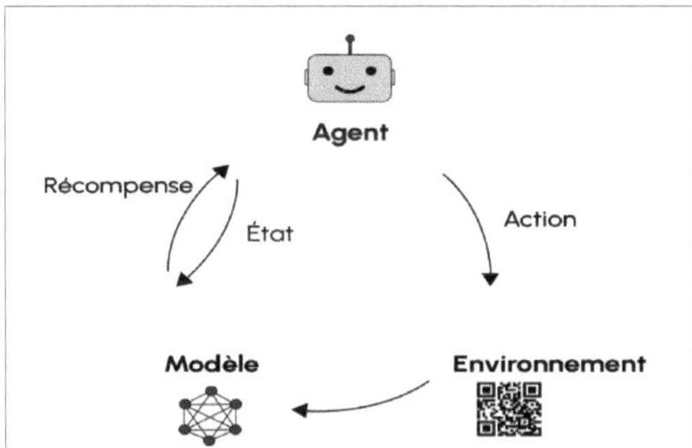

Figure 3: Reinforcement learning scheme [16].

- **Agent:** The learning system.
- **Action**: The actions that the agent can take in response to its environment.
- **Environment:** The environment in which the agent interacts.
- **Model:** The model is used by the agent to make informed decisions about what actions to take. It represents the way in which the agent perceives and understands the environment.

• **Reward / state:** The reward is the signal used by the agent to evaluate the quality of its actions. State represents the current situation in the environment, which can change depending on the agent's actions.

In reinforcement learning, an agent interacts with an environment and makes decisions based on an internal model. It selects and executes actions and receives rewards or penalties depending on its actions. This iterative process is therefore goal- or task-oriented. It allows the agent to learn and improve its performance over time, by taking the best actions, so as to maximise the reward and achieve its specific goals. On the other hand, a task can be episodic or continuous. Episodic tasks have a starting point and an end state, while continuous tasks are those that have no end state, i.e. the agent will run continuously until it is explicitly stopped **[16].** In recent years, AR has seen many new applications, in robotics, the oil industry and bioinformatics **[17]**. The results obtained often exceed human performance, particularly in environments where the action space is discrete, i.e. an environment where the agent has a countable and limited set of actions to undertake.

A concrete example of the application of AR in the healthcare field could be represented by a decision support system for doctors in the choice of treatments **[15]**. The agent would be the AI system that analyses the patient's data and proposes treatment options. The environment would be the patient's specific clinical case, and the actions would be the different treatment options available. The AR system would then learn to adjust the recommendations based on the results observed in previous patients, aimed at optimising medical outcomes **[15]**.

2.3.4. Multi-agent reinforcement learning

Learning by reinforcement learning, in Multi-Agent Reinforcement Learning (MARL) is a field of artificial intelligence and machine learning in which several agents learn to make decisions in a shared or competitive environment. Unlike classical AR where a single agent interacts with the environment, MARL involves multiple agents, each making decisions to achieve its own goals, and these agents can interact with each other and with the environment **[18]**. Key components of MARL include agents taking actions in an environment, states representing the current situation, rewards provided by the environment based on the agents' actions, and challenges related to coordination, competition and cooperation between agents. The algorithms used in MARL aim to enable agents to learn adaptive strategies by taking into account interactions with other agents **[19]**.

3. DEEP LEARNING

3.1. Definition

Around the 20th century[e] , Igor Aizenberg and his colleagues first used the term "deep learning", which was later translated as "apprentissage profond". This discipline is a subset of machine learning, itself part of the wider field of artificial intelligence **[8]**. Deep learning or DL is based on artificial neural networks that mimic the human brain. However, its application requires high computing power for training, as well as large quantities of data to obtain significant results. By analogy with biological neurons, artificial neurons receive input data, perform mathematical operations and then transmit the results to other neurons, forming a complex network until the final result is obtained **[20]**. In short, DL is a powerful method for making complex predictions by mimicking the behaviour of the human brain through the use of artificial neural networks.

3.2. Artificial neural networks

The DL artificial neural networks are organised into three distinct layers, as shown in **Figure 4**.

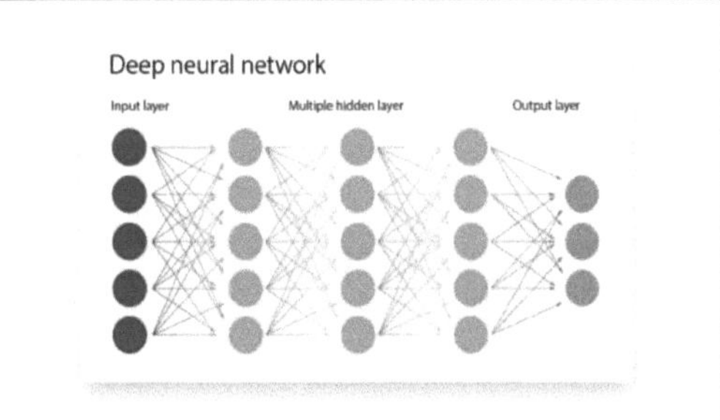

Figure 4: Deep neural network [20].

- The "Input layer" is the layer that receives the initial data.
- The "multiple hidden layer" corresponds to one or more hidden layers that perform complex mathematical calculations on the data.
- The "Output layer" is the output layer. It transmits the final results or predictions of the model for a given problem.

The term "deep" in DL refers to the presence of several hidden layers. One of the major challenges in the design of artificial neural networks lies in the optimal choice of the number of hidden layers and the number of neurons present in each of these layers **[8]**.

Each node, also known as an artificial neuron, establishes connections with other nodes and is characterised by a weight and a threshold. When a node's output exceeds the defined threshold, it is activated and transfers data to the next layer of the network. On the other hand, if the output does not exceed the threshold, no data is transmitted to the next layer **[8]**.

3.3. Algorithms

In deep learning, which is a branch of machine learning, various algorithms are used to train neural network models The company has developed in-depth expertise, particularly in the medical and pharmaceutical fields, to solve specific problems.

Convolutional Neural Networks (CNN) are widely used for image processing and object recognition, particularly in applications such as medical image analysis for tumour detection and organ segmentation **[21]**.

Recursive Neural Networks are used for sequence and natural language processing, enabling the analysis of medical time sequences and the transcription of medical notes **[22]**. Auto-encoders are used for dimension reduction and image generation, facilitating dimension reduction for medical data and the creation of synthetic medical images **[23]**.

Generative Adversarial Networks are essential for the generation of synthetic medical images, data augmentation and medical imaging simulation, for example for microbiome and colonoscopy **[24,25]**. Residual Neural Networks are particularly well suited to training very deep networks for the classification and segmentation of medical images **[26].**

In addition, Transformer Neural Networks are used for natural language processing and contextual understanding models, which are essential for analysing medical texts and extracting clinical information **[27]**.

Short-Term Memory and Long-Term Memory Recurrent Neural Networks are used for modelling sequences and natural language, contributing to the modelling of temporal sequences in the medical field and to the prediction of chronic diseases **[28]**. Finally, Spiking Neural Networks are used to model biologically realistic neurons, providing an accurate simulation of biological neural processes and neural responses **[29]**. In conclusion, all these networks and algorithms could be deployed in various medical and pharmaceutical applications, contributing to significant advances in research, diagnosis, personalised treatment and drug discovery. Their specific use will depend on the particular needs of each task, whether it be the analysis of medical images, the modelling of temporal sequences, or the processing of natural language in the medical context.

3.4. Function cost

In the context of deep learning, the cost function or loss function is a measure that evaluates the difference between the predicted output of the model and the ground truth or real label. Its main objective is to minimise this disparity during model training in order to improve its performance **[30]**.

Several cost functions are available, each tailored to specific types of problem and model output. For example, Mean Square Error is often used for regression tasks, such as predicting numerical values like the effective therapeutic dose of a treatment **[31]**. Binary Cross Entropy is favoured for binary classification tasks, such as detecting the presence or absence of a disease, while Categorical Cross Entropy is adapted to multi-class classification problems, such as classifying distinct diseases **[32]**. Other functions such as "Huber Loss" and "Focal Loss" are also used respectively for robustness to outliers in regression and to deal with class imbalance in classification tasks, often encountered in medical datasets **[30]**.

The specific application of these cost functions in the healthcare field depends on the specific needs of each task. The objective is to judiciously adapt the cost function to the particular nature of the problem to be solved, in order to optimise the model's performance.

4. INTELLIGENCE ARTIFICIAL

4.1. History

The origins of artificial intelligence (AI) date back to the 1950s, when a mathematician named Alan Turing tried to determine whether a machine could show signs of consciousness **[33]**. In his famous article entitled In his book "Computing Machinery and Intelligence", this pioneer in the exploration of this new notion laid the foundations of A and proposed an eponymous test, which he described as an "imitation game", in which a person had to determine whether they were interacting with a human or a machine. Although controversial, the Turing test remained a benchmark in the field of AI **[33]**. In 1965, Edward Feigenbaum (an expert in programming languages), Joshua Lederberg (winner of the Nobel Prize for Medicine) and Carl Djerassi (chemist and inventor of the contraceptive pill) joined forces to create one of the first expert systems in the field of molecular chemistry, which they named DENDRAL "Dendritic Algorithm" in reference to the dendrites of human neurons. This system specialised in interpreting mass spectrometry data to identify the chemical structures of organic molecules **[33]**. The principle of this system was to encapsulate knowledge in the form of rules and facts and to use this knowledge by means of an inference mechanism to solve a problem. This concept was then called "Knowledge Engineering. In 1972, another expert system called MYCIN was born. Designed by Edward H. Shortliffe, the latter focused on the diagnosis of infectious blood diseases, and later meningitis, as well as the prescription of antibiotics **[33]**. MYCIN was equipped with an inference engine similar to that of the DENDRAL system, designed to logically reflect human reasoning. This engine generated highly expert answers by processing the input data. Today, the inference engine continues to be used in various expert systems and AI applications to analyse data and generate logical conclusions based on predefined rules. On the other hand, the Deep Blue supercomputer designed by the American multinational IBM "International Business Machines Corporation" managed to beat the world chess champion Garry Kasparov in 1996 **[34]**. This machine had previously absorbed hundreds of thousands of games played by the greatest masters in the history of chess. It was capable of calculating 200 million moves per second. It was only in 2010 that AI took off again with the emergence of the "This renaissance has also been stimulated by advances in computing capacity and computer storage. This renaissance has also been stimulated by advances in computing and computer storage capacity. **Figure 5** summarises the development of artificial intelligence throughout history.

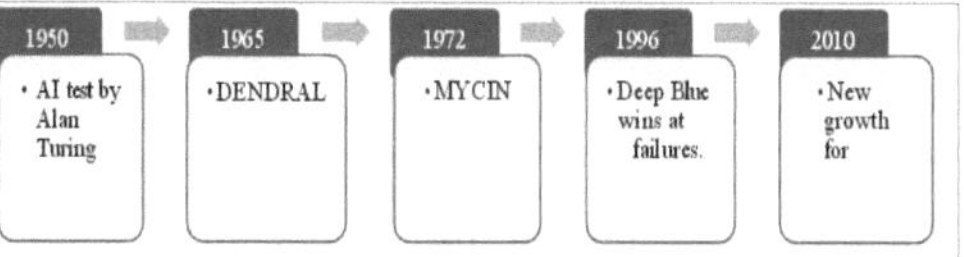

Figure 5: Exploring the historical development of artificial intelligence

AI: Artificial Intelligence

4.2. Definition

In 1956, the American scientist Marvin Lee Minsky defined AI as "the construction of computer programs that perform tasks that are, for the time being, more satisfactorily accomplished by human beings because they require high-level mental processes such as perceptual learning, memory organisation and critical reasoning" **[35]**. According to the European Parliament, AI is any tool used by a machine to "reproduce human-related behaviours, such as reasoning, planning and creativity" **[36]** .

AI can also be defined as a set of techniques designed to enable computers to simulate and reproduce human intelligence. At the heart of AI are algorithms capable of adapting their calculations to suit the tasks at hand. These algorithms are often implemented within artificial neural networks (**Figure 6**), using powerful computing resources to process huge amounts of data and perform complex calculations **[36]**.

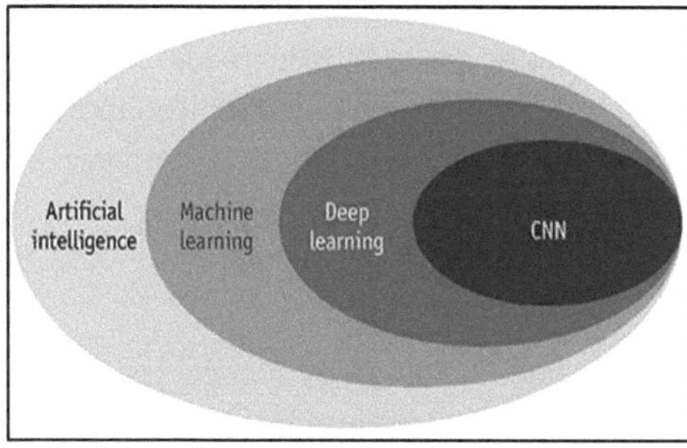

Figure 6: Diagram of the artificial intelligence hierarchy [37].

AI is a broad field that includes multiple techniques such as Machine Learning, which in turn includes more specific methods such as Deep Learning and Convolutional Neural Networks. The latter have a specific architecture of deep neural networks. They are particularly effective for visual perception and image processing, adapted to tasks such as image classification and object detection **(37)**. In addition, AI requires a specialised hardware and software base to write and train machine learning algorithms. No programming language No single language is synonymous with AI, but Python, R, Java, C++ and Julia are the main choices for computer science developers **[37]**.

4.3. State of the art in artificial intelligence

Some AI-related technologies have been around for over 50 years, but advances in computing power, access to vast amounts of data and the development of new algorithms have led to the emergence of AI in recent years. Although its future applications promise significant changes, AI is already playing a crucial role in our daily lives.

4.3.1. Uses outside the healthcare sector

Over the years, artificial intelligence has become increasingly integrated into different aspects of our daily lives, such as digital assistants, intelligent climate control systems, connected objects, autonomous cars, cyber security systems and many other sectors. As a result, AI has grown exponentially in today's market, attracting more and more users and industries. According to forecasts, the AI market is expected to exceed $13 billion by 2026 **[38]**.

4.3.1.1. Autonomous cars

One of the new inventions that various companies such as Tesla, Google and Uber have invested in are autonomous cars. These are a combination of cameras, sensors and AI algorithms that can navigate roads and traffic without human intervention. Autonomous cars have the potential to improve road safety, reduce traffic congestion and increase accessibility for people with disabilities or reduced mobility **[39]** .

4.3.1.2. Digital assistants

At the same time, international technology companies such as Microsoft, IBM, Google and Amazon had been working intensively for several years on the development of new technologies. decades to improve AI-based digital assistants and have recently adapted them for the mass market. Thanks to recent advances in AI, these assistants are now part of our daily lives. We are seeing increasing use of various digital assistants, for example voice assistants such as Amazon Alexa, or text assistants, also known as "These include chatbots such as ChatGPT, launched in November 2022 by OpenAI, and Bard, launched by

Google in July 2023 **[40]** . AI-based digital assistants are expected to become a key part of the future of work. Current business communication platforms, such as Slack or Microsoft Teams, already offer many types of bots to help with day-to-day activities.

4.3.1.3. Marketing

In marketing, AI is used in data collection and analysis processes, the automatic processing of natural language, and so on.
"Today, AI technologies are being used more widely than ever to generate content, improve the customer experience and deliver more accurate results. Today, AI technologies are being used more widely than ever to generate content, improve the customer experience and deliver more accurate results. Botco.ai, a cloud chat communications company using generative AI, conducted an industry research study in March 2023. Surveying 1,000 marketing professionals from over 16 different industries ranging in size from 1 to over 5,000 employees, the results showed that 73% of respondents already use generative AI to help them create text, images, videos or other content**[41]** .

4.3.1.4. Education

The use of AI technologies to simulate teachers' knowledge and experience to provide learners with personalised support or advice has been recognised as a potential solution**[42]** . In In a study carried out in Taiwan in 2020 on primary school pupils, a team of researchers examined the effects of an expert system that took into account both the affective and cognitive status of learners on their results in mathematics **[43]**. The results showed that pupils in the experimental group outperformed those in the other two groups in terms of mathematical achievement. Similarly, this adaptive learning model with analysis of affective and cognitive performance proved more effective in reducing anxiety in these learners.

4.3.2. Use in the health sector

It is well known that AI has made significant contributions to the fields of medicine and pharmacy, with applications ranging from diagnosis and treatment to drug discovery and clinical trials. Indeed, AI-powered tools have provided invaluable assistance to doctors and pharmacists in analysing patient data, identifying potential health risks and developing personalised treatment plans. This has not only led to better health outcomes for patients, but has also accelerated the development of innovative therapies based on new technologies.

4.3.2.1. Diagnosis

AI can transform and simplify many aspects of healthcare, including the diagnostic process. ML, by exploiting data as a primary resource with accuracy dependent on both the quantity and quality of input data, is proving invaluable in tackling the complexities inherent in diagnosis **[44]** . Similarly, it aims to streamline decision-making, optimise workflows and automate tasks efficiently and cost-effectively. In addition, the integration of deep learning, using CNNs and data mining techniques, introduces additional layers capable of discerning complex data patterns. These are widely applicable in healthcare systems, particularly in the identification, prediction and classification of diseases in large datasets **[44]**.

4.3.2.2. Image analysis

In recent years, the spectacular advances made by AI in the analysis of complex images have been propelled by the development of deep learning techniques and the expansion of computing power. Indeed, AI has been used in the interpretation of radiological images, with a particular focus on histopathology and microscopic images of tissue samples. However, it should be noted that cytopathology remains at the top of the pathology fields where AI models for clinical use have been successfully commercialised **[45]**. This distinction underlines the crucial importance of AI in transforming medical practice, paving the way for early detection, accurate diagnosis and effective treatment.

4.3.2.3. Personalised medicine

The advent of AI has revolutionised the field of personalised treatments by offering powerful tools for analysing complex data, predicting outcomes and optimising therapeutic strategies. This pioneering approach has embodied the potential of large-scale precision medicine **[46]**.

One of the pillars of this approach is the ability to provide real-time recommendations, based on advances in machine learning algorithms. These enable patients likely to benefit from specific treatments to be identified on the basis of their genomic profile **[47]**. The key to this personalisation lies in the preliminary genotyping of patients, making it possible to anticipate their needs and adapt drugs and dosages accordingly. This proactive approach paves the way for more precise and effective medicine, offering new prospects for improving patient health **[47]**.

4.3.2.4. Helping to optimise chemotherapy

Current practice in chemotherapy is to give patients the maximum tolerated dose. Although this approach aims to maximise the effectiveness of the treatment, it does not always succeed in achieving this objective and is often accompanied by significant side effects, adversely affecting patients' quality of life. Faced with these limitations, A. Balsiak and his team have developed CURATE.AI, an innovative AI-based platform that dynamically adjusts chemotherapy doses based on data specific to each patient **[48]**. The platform generates personalised doses for treatment cycles by analysing the correlation between variations in chemotherapy doses and tumour markers **[48]**. Their prospective open-label study also showed that the integration of CURATE.AI into the clinical workflow proved successful, highlighting potential benefits in terms of reduced chemotherapy doses, improved patient response rates and response times compared to standard treatments **[48]**. These encouraging results underline the need for further research through randomised clinical trials to validate the efficacy of this tool. They also pave the way for more widespread use of AI in the field of chemotherapy dose optimisation, with the aim of reducing the risk of adverse drug reactions and improving patients' quality of life.

4.4. Regulatory and ethical aspects

The last few years have seen remarkable growth and acceptance of AI in various fields, particularly among healthcare professionals. AI offers rich opportunities for designing intelligent products, creating innovative services and generating new business models. However, its use can also raise social and ethical challenges in terms of security, confidentiality and human rights. The integration of AI technologies into practical, safe and effective healthcare applications, services and procedures involves significant costs and risks, underlining the importance of protecting the commercial interests associated with these technologies **[49]**. It is imperative to take into account the ethical risks associated with the implementation of AI in healthcare, particularly with regard to the violation of privacy and data confidentiality, informed consent and patient autonomy. In a context where AI is playing a crucial role in healthcare, robust data protection legislation is needed to safeguard patient privacy. In this regard, laws such as the US law that establishes data privacy requirements for organisations responsible for safeguarding protected patient data HIPAA "Health Insurance Portability and Accountability Act" and the General Data Protection Regulation (GDPR) in Europe have been put in place to protect personal data **[50]**. However, HIPAA has significant shortcomings in the current healthcare context, as it only covers specific health information. It is therefore not sufficient to protect patient health privacy in the United States **[49]**. The GDPR, on the other hand, is a European Union law that came into force in 2018 to protect individuals' personal data. It applies to any business operating in the EU, including in some situations, those located outside the territory **[50]**. Unlike HIPAA in the US, the GDPR is broader and covers a wide range of personal health data. It prohibits the processing of certain special categories of data, such as genetic data, unless they meet strict criteria defined by law **[50]**. The GDPR also includes provisions relevant to the integration of AI in medicine, requiring in particular a data protection impact assessment for new AI-based technologies **[50]**.

Another regulatory aspect to consider in the application of artificial intelligence in healthcare is standards of evidence. These are criteria or requirements established by regulatory authorities or healthcare bodies to assess the effectiveness, safety and reliability of medical technologies, including those based on AI **[51]**. They define the thresholds with which products or technologies must comply in order to be authorised for use in medical practice. For example, for AI applications involved in medical prediction, diagnosis and treatment, the standards of evidence must be significantly higher than for imaging applications using AI **[51]**. Ensuring that these standards are adequately defined and kept up to date is a major challenge for regulatory and public health bodies. It is therefore essential to strike a balance between promoting innovation and protecting patients from these potential risks, while preserving their right to privacy and data security.

4.5.The limits of artificial intelligence in healthcare

The use of AI in healthcare has a number of limitations that must be taken into account to ensure its effectiveness and safety.

4.5.1. The data

There are many data-related challenges in the field of AI in healthcare. On the one hand, the scarcity of patient data is a major barrier to global research, as real data is often protected by privacy laws **[52]**. The sharing and use of medical data is sensitive and raises important ethical and legal issues, including patient consent and privacy. On the other hand, clinical data is often noisy, containing incomplete or erroneous information, requiring considerable time to make it usable **[52]**. Indeed, the use of non-standardised data can lead to erroneous predictions or inaccurate clinical decisions. In addition, adversarial cyber attacks, which aim to manipulate data or AI models to produce erroneous results, pose a serious threat to the reliability of healthcare AI systems **[52]**. These challenges highlight the need to develop robust strategies for data collection, cleansing and protection in healthcare to ensure safe and reliable applications.

4.5.2. The black box of artificial intelligence

In the field of machine learning, CNNs are widely used tools for processing complex data, such as medical images. However, a major challenge with these models is their "black box" nature, in other words their lack of transparency in the way they adjust their internal parameters, such as the weights assigned to each neural connection and the learning rate **[53]**. This opacity makes it difficult to understand how the model makes its decisions, which is particularly critical in the field of health, where the reliability and explicability of models are essential. Indeed, understanding how models make decisions is crucial to clinicians' and patients' confidence in their use. Consequently, it is necessary to develop methods to make the learning and decision-making processes of CNN models more transparent and comprehensible, in order to guarantee their effective and reliable use in medical applications.

4.5.3. Biases

The presence of biases in AI data and algorithms can lead to disparities in clinical outcomes and increase health inequalities. It is therefore important to detect and correct these biases to ensure equitable healthcare **[54]**.

Here are some examples of the most common biases:

- **Data selection bias:** This type of bias occurs when the data used to train an algorithm does not fairly represent the target population. For example, if the data used to develop a diagnostic model does not include diverse patient subgroups, this can lead to biased results that are not generalizable to the population as a whole (54).
- **Social class bias:** Health data can often reflect socio-economic disparities, which can introduce bias into the results of algorithms. For example, if the data used to predict clinical outcomes are based primarily on high-income populations, this may lead to treatment recommendations that are not suitable for people on lower incomes (54).

- **Race and ethnicity bias:** AI algorithms can also reproduce racial and ethnic biases present in training data. If the data used to develop an algorithm is biased towards certain racial or ethnic groups, this can lead to discriminatory results that are not fair or equitable **[55]** .
- **Gender bias:** Health data can also be influenced by gender bias, which can lead to unfair treatment recommendations for men and women. For example, if the data used to train a heart disease prediction model is based primarily on men, this may lead to missed diagnoses in women **[56]**.
- **Algorithmic bias:** AI algorithms themselves can be biased, either because of the way they are designed or because of the data on which they are trained. If an algorithm is designed to favour certain results over others, this can lead to unfair or inequitable treatment recommendations (54).

4.5.4. Public perception

Public perception can be a major limitation to the widespread adoption of AI. Individuals' attitudes and beliefs towards AI, whether in terms of its potential to replace or assist healthcare professionals, its impact on the quality of care or the level of trust placed in these systems, can greatly influence its acceptance and integration. In addition, studies have shown that health preferences can vary according to cultural, social and demographic contexts, highlighting the importance of a thorough understanding of the general public's perceptions for the successful implementation of AI in healthcare **[57]** . In short, although this technology offers promising possibilities in the field of healthcare, its limitations must be addressed proactively to maximise its benefits while minimising its potential risks. The recent WHO publication stresses the crucial importance of ensuring the safety and effectiveness of AI systems in healthcare, as well as the need to foster collaboration between the various stakeholders, including technology developers, regulators, manufacturers, medical practitioners and healthcare recipients **[58]** .

5. APPLICATIONS OF ARTIFICIAL INTELLIGENCE

In this section, we have explored some recent clinical studies that illustrate the application of artificial intelligence in the medical and pharmaceutical fields in order to highlight how AI has revolutionised modern medicine, whether in computer-assisted diagnosis, prediction of medical outcomes, drug discovery or adverse event monitoring. We also detail the crucial support provided by AI during the COVID-19 crisis and its essential role in predicting the viral structure of Sars-Cov-2. The examples chosen will attempt to demonstrate how advances in AI continue to transform medical and pharmaceutical practices, opening up new possibilities for improving public health and the well-being of society.

5.1. Applications in the medical field

5.1.1. Medical imaging

5.1.1.1. Pelvic ultrasound

Ultrasound is a flexible imaging modality used worldwide as a first-line medical examination procedure and in many different clinical cases. It benefits from the continuous evolution of ultrasound technologies and from a well-established ultrasound-based digital healthcare system. Nevertheless, its diagnostic performance is still problematic due to the inherent characteristics of ultrasound imaging, such as manual operation and heavy dependence on the operator. Multiple studies have already shown that AI is capable of recognising complex scanning patterns and providing quantitative assessments of imaging data. This technology can therefore help doctors to obtain more accurate and reproducible ultrasound results **[59]**. According to Fiorentino et al, 3D ultrasound is widely used for its ability to provide rich spatial and diagnostic information, which is difficult to obtain with 2D ultrasound **[60]**. In addition, it allows multiple standard planes (SPs) to be captured in a single shot. However, manual localisation of SPs in 3D ultrasound is difficult due to low image quality, huge search space and high anatomical variability. To address this challenge, Fiorentino's team proposed a novel MARL learning framework that automatically locates multiple PSs in 3D pelvic ultrasound. This approach not only improved user independence, but also increased scanning efficiency. Thus, the proposed method was a robust approach that accurately locates multiple PSs in different datasets, in this case pelvic ultrasounds **[60]**.

In addition, the researchers have combined a MARL system with a Recursive Neural Network to form a collaborative module that enhances communication,

information sharing, joint decision-making and concerted action between agents. The aim of this combined system is to efficiently localise several SPs in 3D ultrasound scans. The researchers adopted neural architecture research to automatically design the architecture of the agent network and the collaborative module **[60]**. In other words, they applied machine learning techniques to determine the optimal configuration of the neural network used by the agents and the collaborative module, rather than defining this structure manually.
The results of their study showed that a MARL-type ML model enables the automatic and efficient localisation of PS on pelvic ultrasound scans from normal and abnormal uteri. This AI-based method is therefore applicable in a variety of clinical contexts.

5.1.1.2. Chest X-rays

The application of AI to chest X-rays can be illustrated by the work of Tayebi Arasteh et al. who examined the use of self-supervised learning (SSL) for pre-training AI models to analyse medical images, in particular chest X-rays **[61]**.
In the field of advanced medical image analysis, it has become common practice to use datasets in which images have previously been labelled. These labels are pieces of information associated with each image that indicate what the image represents, for example, the presence or absence of certain medical conditions.
While pre-labelled datasets have become a technical standard in the analysis of medical images using AI, the emergence of SSL offers an opportunity to bypass the intensive labelling process. It is therefore an intermediate technique between supervised and unsupervised learning.
Figure 7 highlights the process and benefits of using SSL as a pre-training method for AI models in medical imaging analysis.
In **step (a)**, supervised learning demonstrates the traditional AI pre-training process using labelled datasets, which can be resource and time intensive due to the need for manual annotation.
The SSL method in **step (b)** involves training AI models on non-medical, unlabelled images, taking advantage of freely available data, thus bypassing the costly and time-consuming need for manual labelling. Finally, in **step (c)**, the transfer of knowledge acquired from the SSL pre-trained model on non-medical images to a supervised model enables medical images to be diagnosed accurately.

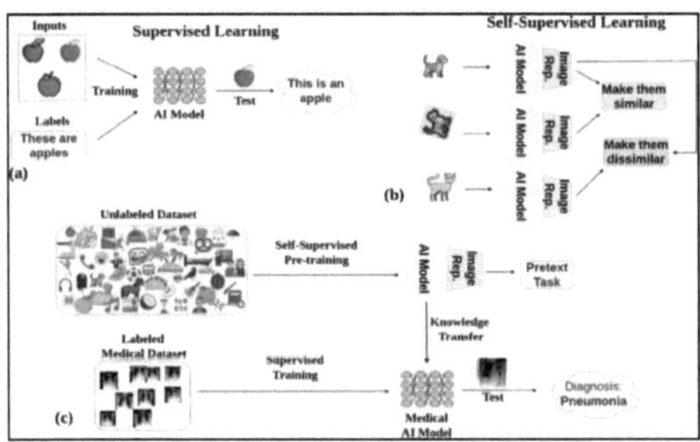

Figure 7: Difference between supervised and self-supervised learning [61].

As mentioned earlier in supervised learning, the training data is labelled, which means that each example of data is associated with a label that indicates the correct response. The model is trained to predict these labels from the input data provided. In unsupervised learning, the training data is not labelled. The model has to find meaningful structures or groupings in this data on its own, without any external supervision. SSL represents an ML approach where a model acquires knowledge from unlabelled data by defining its own supervisory tasks. In this process, the algorithm divides the data into distinct segments, using some to generate predictions and others to evaluate them. This process allows the algorithm to improve incrementally without the need for initial supervision **[61]**.
In this study, Tayebi Arasteh's team wanted to examine whether pre-training with SSL on large databases of unannotated images, can improve the performance of medical AI models compared to pre-training with supervised learning. They tested this approach by training AI models to diagnose more than 20 radiological imaging results on a multisite dataset covering three continents and comprising more than 800,000 chest X-rays. The researchers compared the performance of the SSL method with that of the supervised model on non-medical images from the ImageNet database and on labelled chest X-rays from the MIMIC-CXR database **[61]**.
The results showed that the performance of SSL not only outperformed the initial training phase of the supervised model based on non-medical images, but in some cases also outperformed the supervised model on labelled chest X-rays. These results suggest that the choice of initial training strategy may be crucial for improving the diagnostic accuracy of artificial intelligence in medical imaging **[61]**. In the context of medical diagnosis, SSL represents a paradigm shift towards improving the accuracy and efficiency of AI models. This study highlights the importance of further exploring the application of self-supervised

learning in medical imaging, particularly in contexts where exhaustively labelled datasets are limited.

5.1.2. Medical diagnosis

5.1.2.1. Diagnosis of autism

An example of the application of AI in the medical diagnosis of autism is highlighted by Kim et al. through the development of "deep ensemble models" to differentiate retinal photographs of people with autism spectrum disorders (ASD) from people with typical development (TD) **[62]**. This The ensemblistic model also allows a distinction to be made between cases of severe ASD and mild to moderate ASD.

Kim et al. conducted a diagnostic study in a hospital in Seoul, South Korea, on 958 participants with a mean age of 8 years **[62]**. Retinal photographs of individuals with ASD were collected prospectively, and those of age- and sex-matched individuals with TD were collected retrospectively. The neural network used to build these ensemblistic models is a pre-trained ResNeXt-50 network. This is a specific type of deep CNN network architecture. By using a pre-trained network, the set models can benefit from the knowledge previously acquired by the network on a large amount of data. This can often speed up and improve the learning process when applied to new datasets or tasks. All statistical analyses were performed using Python, and all classification models were implemented using the PyTorch library **[62]**.

The results of this study suggest that retinal photographs may be a promising objective method for screening for ASD and even for assessing the severity of symptoms. The AUROC, or 'Area Under the Receiver Operating Characteristic curve', is a measure commonly used in ML and diagnostic testing to assess the performance of a binary classification model. The mean AUROC values for ASD screening and symptom severity were 1.00 and 0.74 respectively. A high AUROC value, close to 1, indicates that the model has good discriminative capacity, i.e. it can effectively distinguish individuals with ASD from those without. In addition, the ASD screening models were able to provide very accurate predictions when confronted with data similar to that on in which they had been trained. Thus, the predictions of the models were very close to reality, indicating estimates with good accuracy **[62]**. The models used also showed promising results in distinguishing ASD from TD based on retinal photographs, suggesting that retinal alterations associated with ASD could serve as potential biomarkers. The models maintained a mean AUROC of 1.00 using only 10% of the image containing the optic disc, highlighting the crucial importance of this

area in distinguishing ASD from TD. The results also suggest that retinal photographs could be used as an objective screening tool from at least 4 years of age. However, according to the authors, this does not mean that retinal photographs are not feasible for children under 4 years of age, and further research in this direction is essential **[62]**.
In summary, the AI was able to differentiate children with ASD from children with TD, and even when 90% of the non-critical areas of the images were removed, the models maintained perfect performance. This research represents a significant advance towards the development of objective screening tools for ASDs, which could potentially help solve the problems of access to specialist child psychiatry assessments due to limited resources.

5.1.2.2. Diagnosis of depression

In 2023, the US company Aiberry Inc created a multimodal AI platform that analyses facial, audio and text features to screen for mental disorders **[63]**. A group of professors and students at Oxford University and the University of Paris hypothesised 15 years ago that depression could be detected by analysing our unique facial muscles. This hypothesis has evolved to take account of the knowledge available from contextual analysis of voice and words. The Conventional measures of depression, such as the Beck, Zung or Carroll scales, require individuals to self-assess the frequency and severity of their depressive symptoms by selecting the response that best describes them from a series of multiple-choice questions **[64]**. Aiberry's app offers an innovative AI-based assessment option, featuring a digital animation called Botberry that encourages users to talk about themselves in their own words. Machine learning software aggregates the responses to these questions and generates an overall depression risk score, as well as symptom-level information and a transcript of each response **[63]**.
Similarly, a rigorous study conducted by the University of Texas at Austin demonstrated that the Aiberry application was clinically equivalent to the "gold standard" in mental health assessment **[63]**. Its main objective was to use a demographically diverse sample to validate an AI model, previously trained on interviews administered by humans, on new interviews administered by robots, and to check for algorithmic biases linked to criteria such as age, gender, race and ethnicity **[63]**.
Around 400 adults were recruited via social networks to take part in a brief interview administered by a robot and completed a depression self-assessment form. An AI model was used to predict form scores based solely on interview responses. For any significant discrepancies between the model interpretation

and the form score, clinicians conducted a masked review to determine which they preferred **[63]**.

The results showed a strong and positive correlation between the model's predictions and self-reported scores, with a correlation coefficient r of 0.73 and a mean absolute error of 3.3. Indeed, 90% of AI predictions were in agreement with self-report or clinical expert opinion when The AI contradicted the self-assessment. There was no difference in model performance according to age, sex, race or ethnic origin **[63]**. Thus, this study demonstrates that AI can accurately predict the severity of depression based on oral responses collected remotely during an interview conducted by a robot. These results are promising for the use of this technology as a mental health screening tool to help clinicians in clinical decision-making.

5.1.2.3. Diagnosis of diabetic retinopathy

In August 2020, EyeNuk Inc, an international AI-based medical technology and services company, became the leader in eye screening with the launch of the EyeArt system, which has been approved by the US Food and Drug Administration (FDA) **[65]**. The system identifies more than mild diabetic retinopathy (mtmDR) and vision-threatening diabetic retinopathy. It has been approved as a class IIb medical device in the European Union to identify DR, glaucomatous optic nerve damage and age-related macular degeneration in a single test.

In a recent publication involving more than 500 trial participants, Lim et al. aimed to compare the diagnostic performance of ophthalmologists and the EyeArt AI system for the detection of mtmDR **[65]**. Patients over 18 years of age with diabetes and no history of DR who could tolerate a fundus were eligible. Participants underwent several retinal photographs for analysis by the artificial AI system. The results were compared with dilated ophthalmoscopy methods for detecting DR in diabetic patients. The results of this study showed that the EyeArt AI system had a higher sensitivity for detecting mtmDR compared with dilated ophthalmoscopy: 96.4% for EyeArt ($CI_{95\%}$ = [93.1%-99.8%]) compared with 27.7% for ophthalmoscopy ($CI_{95\%}$ = [20.1-35.2%]). However, its specificity was slightly lower: 88.4% compared with 99.6% **[65]**.

Thus, we can consider EyeArt as an interesting screening tool with its high sensitivity for the detection of mtmDR. Unlike human-based tele-screening systems, the EyeArt system provides an immediate determination of the presence of mtmDR that is available to the patient before leaving the primary care practice, thereby improving adherence to follow-up care. In addition, it represents the first FDA-cleared autonomous diagnostic AI system in any field of medicine, with the potential to help prevent vision loss in thousands of people with diabetes each year.

5.1.3. Disease prediction

5.1.3.1. Prediction of pancreatic cancer

Pancreatic cancer is an aggressive disease with a poor prognosis that is often diagnosed late, so it needs to be detected as early as possible. In this context, collaborative work between Harvard Medical School and the University of Copenhagen has revealed that an artificial intelligence tool has been able to effectively identify, up to three years before diagnosis, people at high risk of pancreatic cancer, based solely on patients' medical records **[66]**. In fact, the researchers developed an AI model based on combinations of disease codes and their "timing" of appearance, which enabled them to predict which patients are likely to develop pancreatic cancer in the future. These combinations of disease codes could include sequences of medical diagnoses associated with an increased risk of pancreatic cancer. For example, the presence of unspecified jaundice followed by pancreatic problems could indicate pancreatic dysfunction associated with a risk of pancreatic cancer. Similarly, the diagnosis of type 2 diabetes followed by unspecified gastrointestinal problems could indicate an increased susceptibility to this type of cancer in diabetic patients. In addition, the presence of gallstones accompanied by persistent abdominal pain could indicate irritation or obstruction of the pancreas, thereby increasing the risk of cancer **[66]**.

In this study, the researchers tested different versions of the AI models to detect people at high risk of developing the disease in different time frames of 6 months, one year, 2 years and 3 years. Each version of the algorithm proved to be much more accurate than current estimates of the incidence of the disease in the population, with a capacity comparable to current genetic sequencing tests. To assess the risk of pancreatic cancer, they used recently developed ML predictive models using patient records from a variety of sources such as health surveys, GP registers and real-world hospital databases. Rather than simply identifying disease already present, their approach allowed the evolution of disease over time to be taken into account, providing a more dynamic and detailed perspective for predicting pancreatic cancer risk **[66]**.

One of the main advantages of this AI tool is that it can be used on all patients for whom medical records are available, allowing early detection in high-risk individuals who may not be aware of their genetic predisposition or family history. By using this tool, clinicians could target the right populations for more advanced testing, while avoiding unnecessary additional tests and procedures for others. In addition, this tool represents a critical first step in improving screening, targeted testing and early diagnosis of pancreatic cancer, offering a valuable opportunity to save lives.

5.1.3.2. Prediction of COVID-19 mortality

In October 2020, Gao et al. presented a mortality risk prediction model for COVID-19, which they named the Mortality Risk Prediction Ensemble Model (MRPMC) **[67]**. This model uses clinical data from patients with COVID-19 on admission to stratify patients according to mortality risk, making it possible to predict physiological deterioration and death up to 20 days in advance **[67]**. MRP? is a set model, which allows it to capture a variety of structures and relationships in the data, improving its predictive ability. It was built using four machine learning methods, including logistic regression, support vector machine, gradient boosted decision tree and neural network **[67]**. This mortality risk prediction model has been validated in several validation cohorts. Thus, it offered a promising approach to improving the management of patients with COVID-19 by enabling accurate prediction of mortality risk and facilitating a more proactive and tailored medical response.

Several other researchers have used ML and DL to predict the status of patients with COVID-19. In April 2023, Qiu-Yu Li et al. used ML to detect severe early clinical warning signals in patients with COVID-19 **[68]**. In a comprehensive study published in March 2023, Jin et al. also used DL in COVID-19 research **[69]**. They concluded that this tool has the potential not only to diagnose COVID-19, but also to judge the progression and prognosis of the disease, suggest treatment plans and help health authorities formulate intelligent measures to control and prevent the spread of the disease.

5.2. Pharmaceutical applications

5.2.1. Discovery of antibiotics

Since the discovery of penicillin, antibiotics have been an essential part of modern medicine. However, the continued effectiveness of these vital remedies is being called into question by the emergence of multi-resistant strains. This problem is further exacerbated by the decline in the development of new molecules, a phenomenon attributable to a lack of economic incentives. Faced with this alarming situation, the search for new antibiotics is becoming

increasingly complex. To meet this challenge, new approaches to antibiotic discovery are needed to increase the rate of identification of new molecules and, at the same time, reduce the costs associated with their early discovery. Fortunately, recent advances in machine learning are paving the way for the application of algorithms for the prediction of molecular properties, enabling the identification of new structural classes of antibiotics **[70]**. Unlike traditional high-throughput screening methods, which limit their tests to a few million molecules, contemporary algorithmic approaches can evaluate hundreds of millions or even billions of molecules for their antibacterial properties. This ability to explore vast chemical spaces far exceeds the scope of current experimental approaches **[70]**.
On the other hand, antimicrobial resistance represents a major threat on a global scale for the health, social, environmental and economic sectors, requiring sustained action to remedy it. The development of antimicrobial resistance complicates the treatment of infections, increases the spread of disease, its severity and the risk of death. As a result, the effectiveness of medicines diminishes, allowing infections to persist in the body and increasing the risk of transmission to other individuals.

5.2.1.1. Development of Halicine

In a recent study published in 2020, AI researchers Stokes et al. aimed to demonstrate how the combination of in silico predictions and empirical laboratory investigations can lead to the discovery of new antibiotics **[70]**. Their approach consisted of three stages. First, they trained a deep neural network model to predict Escherichia coli growth inhibition using a collection of 2335 molecules. This model works by constructing a molecular graph based on a specific property, in this case E. coli growth inhibition, using a message-passing approach, iteratively exchanging information about the local chemistry between adjacent atoms and bonds in a series of message-passing steps. Each iteration propagates the local chemistry information throughout the molecule, allowing the model to build a more holistic representation of the molecule. After a defined number of message-passing steps, the vector representations of the different local chemical regions of a molecule are summed into a single continuous vector that captures the complexity of the whole compound. They then applied the resulting model to several separate chemical libraries, comprising more than 107 million molecules, to identify potential compounds with activity against this germ. After ranking the compounds according to the score predicted by the model, they finally selected a list of candidate molecules

based on a predefined prediction score threshold, chemical structure and availability **[70]**.
In this work, the scientists reported that they initially identified 99 distinct molecules within the "Drug Repurposing Hub", a database that compiles a variety of chemical compounds, mainly drugs already approved for other clinical indications. These molecules were the most strongly predicted by the AI model to have antibacterial properties, and were then subjected to empirical testing to assess their ability to inhibit the growth of E. coli. Of these compounds, 51 demonstrated growth inhibition against the germ. These molecules were then ranked according to their stage ofclinical investigation, their structural similarity to the molecules in the main training set, and their predicted toxicity using a deep neural network model trained on the ClinTox database. The compound that met all these criteria was the c-Jun N-terminal kinase inhibitor SU3327, renamed Halicin **[70]**. Its chemical structure, described in **Figure 8**, corresponds to a nitrothiazole derivative that was previously studied as a potential treatment for diabetes but was not further developed for this application due to poor study results. Halicin demonstrated excellent growth inhibitory activity against E. coli, with a minimum inhibitory concentration of 2 µg/ml.

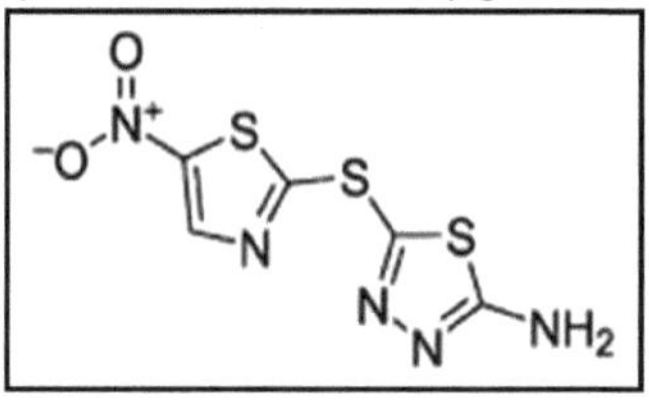

Figure 8: Chemical structure of halicin [70].

Significantly, the researchers found that the prediction rank of halicin in their model (position 89) was higher than that of the other models tested. These data underline the importance of using a message-passing deep neural network approach in the discovery of new antibiotic candidates, such as halicin.

5.2.1.2. Development of Abaucine

Acinetobacter baumannii is an opportunistic bacterium that stands out as a top priority among infectious pathogens, due to its widespread resistance to virtually all classes of antibiotics and available therapeutic modalities. The strain of A. baumannii resistant to carbapenems is categorised as one of the critical priority pathogens on the WHO list of antibiotic-resistant bacteria, requiring urgent efforts to develop effective drugs **[71]**. In addition, A. baumanni is generally found in hospitals, where it can survive on surfaces for long periods. The pathogen is capable of picking up deoxyribonucleic acid from other species of bacteria in its environment, including antibiotic resistance genes.

A retrospective study published in 2021 was carried out in this context in the burns intensive care unit of the Ben Arous Traumatology and Burns Centre in Tunisia **[72]**. The aim was to analyse the incidence densities of A. baumannii colonisation and infection and the antibiotic resistance of strains isolated from hospitalised patients. The results showed that this germ has a high level of resistance to the antibiotics tested, such as ceftazidime, piperacillin-tazobactam and ciprofloxacin. According to a new study published in May 2023 in the scientific journal Nature Chemical Biology, Stokes et al, researchers at McMaster University and the Massachusetts Institute of Technology, used an artificial intelligence algorithm to predict new structural classes of antibacterial molecules and succeeded in identifying a new antibacterial compound effective against the dreaded A. baumannii bacterium **[73]** . They named this new antibiotic Abaucine (**Figure 9**).

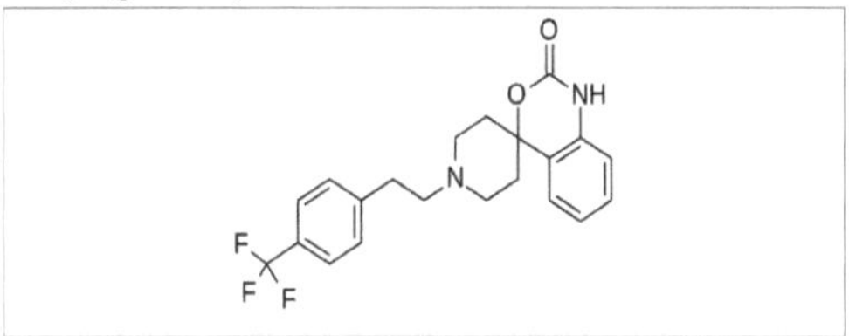

Figure 9: Chemical structure of Abaucine [73].

In order to identify Abaucine, the authors built on their previous work carried out in 2020, which enabled them to demonstrate the usefulness of machine learning in the discovery of new antibacterial molecules using E. coli K12 as a model organism **[70]**. For example, they used a dataset containing molecules with the ability to inhibit the growth of A. baumannii bacteria in vitro, including off-patent drugs and synthetic chemicals selected from various high-throughput screening sub-libraries. They used this data to train a particular type of message-passing neural network, which translates the graphical structure of a molecule into a continuous vector **[73]**. They then used this trained neural network to make predictions on the Drug Repurposing Hub, a database containing nearly 7,500 potential drug molecules. They specifically looked for molecules that were not already known to have activity against A. baumannii, i.e. that had not yet been identified as antibiotics for this bacterium **[73]**. Similarly, the predictions of the trained neural network found a total of 240 priority molecules meeting specific criteria. It should be noted that the model was optimised using a set of ten classifiers, which increased its robustness **[73]**. This approach clearly shows that ML has been integrated at several stages in the process of identifying and validating candidate antibacterial molecules. These molecules were acquired and tested in vitro against A. baumannii at a concentration of 50µM. Using a strict threshold of over 80% growth inhibition, nine of the molecules tested showed antibacterial activity against this germ. Elimination criteria relating to molecular structure were applied to these nine priority molecules, resulting in the selection of a single molecule. Subsequent research focused on this molecule, which was given the name Abaucine. After conducting more experiments with this product to assess bacterial viability after treatment, a modest bactericidal activity was observed **[73]**. After 6 hours of treatment, the researchers withdrew the compound from the A. baumannii cultures and observed a resumption of bacterial growth, with the apparent latency period increasing with increasing concentrations of Abaucine **[73]**. Overall, these data show the antibacterial efficacy of this compound, inhibiting a biological process that was maximally active during growth and division, which is consistent with most known antibiotics.

Secondly, the researchers presented solid evidence that Abaucine possesses narrow-spectrum antibacterial activity, which is advantageous for reducing the inter-pathogenic spread of resistance. In addition, experiments have shown that Abaucine could control A. baumannii infection in a mouse wound model, which means that Abaucine has the potential to reduce or limit infection caused by A. baumannii in a specific animal model, in this case in mice **[73]**. This information is important because it indicates that abaucin has therapeutic potential in the treatment of infections caused by this bacterium.

Finally, this study highlighted the usefulness of machine learning in antibiotic discovery and described a promising lead with targeted activity against a multi-resistant Gram-negative pathogen. The discovery of new antibiotics against A. baumannii using conventional screening has proved difficult. Traditional methods are time-consuming, expensive and limited. Modern algorithmic approaches provide access to hundreds of millions, if not billions, of molecules with antibacterial properties. The process used by these researchers could also accelerate the discovery of other antibiotics to treat many other multi-resistant bacteria. In conclusion, the researchers have responded to the urgent need for new drugs to treat Acinetobacter baumannii, a multi-drug resistant bacterium. a nosocomial bacterium that is difficult to eradicate and can cause pneumonia, meningitis and wound infections, even leading to death.

5.2.2. Fight against Covid-19

The COVID-19 pandemic began to emerge at the end of 2019, with the first cases reported in December in Wuhan, China. It then spread rapidly around the world during 2020, becoming a major global health crisis**[74]** .
Although overwhelmed healthcare institutions sought to mitigate the pandemic, mortality continued to rise. The scientific community has expressed high hopes for the potential of data science and AI to contribute to the fight against the pandemic.

5.2.2.1. Bibliographic research

Since the outbreak of COVID-19, thousands of scientific articles have been published covering various aspects of the disease, from potential treatments to the dynamics of the pandemic, demonstrating the urgency with which researchers have responded to this health crisis. However, this massive influx of scientific literature presented a challenge for anyone wishing to exploit the data to draw relevant conclusions.
To overcome this problem, the White House Office of Science and Technology Policy in the United States asked researchers and managers from the Allen Institute for AI and Emerging Technologies at Georgetown University, Microsoft and the National Library of Medicine to collaborate and create a database compiling the scientific literature on COVID-19, SARS-CoV-2 and coronavirus in general **[75]**. This database, called CORD-19 "COVID-19 Open Research Dataset", brought together publications from PubMed Central, the bioRxiv and medRxiv pre-publication servers, and the WHO database on COVID-19. During the pandemic, CORD-19 was a valuable resource for the development of AI-powered tools and applications. Researchers and
"Data scientists can use this database to train machine learning models, natural language processing algorithms and other AI techniques to extract information, identify trends and develop solutions related to disease research, treatment and prevention. Indeed, analysis of the vast amount of coronavirus data has been facilitated by AI-based research tools such as WellAI and SciSight **[75]**.
The WellAI application uses NLP-type neural networks to learn from the CORD-19 database in order to summarise existing knowledge **[75]**. The main objective of this application is to help researchers generate new ideas or concepts relevant to their research on the virus. Rather than simply providing summaries of existing knowledge, the application uses unsupervised learning to discover new aspects or potential new directions in the data, which can inspire researchers to explore new avenues of research or formulate new hypotheses

[75].Similarly, SciSight is an AI-powered visualisation tool for exploring associations between concepts appearing in the CORD-19 database [75]. These concepts can include medical terms, proteins, genes, diseases, chemicals, and so on. The tool also visualises the emerging network of literature around coronavirus, which means that it provides a graphical representation of the relationships between these concepts in the scientific literature [76]. This allows users to better understand how the different aspects of the disease and its research are interconnected and how they evolve over time. In addition, SciSight is based on SciBERT, a pre-trained language model trained on a large corpus of scientific publications, in order to provide improved performance in NLP [76].
In practice, there are several advantages to using tools that exploit NLP compared to a conventional search engine (**Table II**).

Table II: Comparison of NLP-based machine learning tools and a conventional search engine [75].

	Powered search tool by AI based on NLP	Search engine for classic publications
Objective	Neural networks	Search for keywords and
general	summarise, generalise and	sentences in an article. Cannot
	predict relationships between	not draw any conclusions about the
	key words.	relationships between keywords.
Synonyms	The tool is capable of	Results produced
(concepts	understand synonyms and	correspond to keywords or
correlated)	correlated concepts. For example,	search phrases, without
	he understands that	knowledge of synonyms and
	"Hypertension" is a	associated concepts.
	synonymous with "high blood	
	pressure" and "elevated blood	
	pressure".	
Results	The result is aggregated and summarised,	The result is not aggregated, nor
	this is a structured list of	In short, it's a list of
	concepts with probabilities	each occurrence (i.e.
	classified. This reduces the scope of	each article) of a word or an
	work and increases efficiency	sentence.
	research.	

AI: Artificial Intelligence; NLP: Natural language processing

Let's take the example of a search using the WellAI tool in relation to Pubmed. By specifying the prior concept of "COVID-19" and adding the concept "Clinical Diagnosis", the WellAI results will display a list of articles in which the machine learning models have identified a relationship between the two concepts **[75]**. On the other hand, on Pubmed, a search using the same terms returns a list of all articles mentioning "COVID-19" and "Clinical diagnosis". "clinical diagnosis", without necessarily establishing a link between the two **[75]**. Thus, an article may mention these terms without actually dealing with the subject of clinical diagnosis, as the terms may simply appear in the references section.

5.2.2.2. Vaccine design

One of the most anticipated applications of AI during the pandemic was its use in designing a vaccine to contain the pandemic. In February 2020, the Chinese technology multinational Baidu unveiled a machine-learning algorithm called Linearfold **[77]**. By studying protein folding, this algorithm can predict the structure of viral ribonucleic acid molecules in a record time of 27 seconds, as opposed to the 55 minutes required by conventional algorithms [77]. This advance has provided scientists with crucial information about the spread of the virus. AI has thus made it possible to predict the structure of the virus more quickly and save months of experimental work.In the same context, DeepMind, a subsidiary of Alphabet, also announced in August 2020 its predictions concerning the structure of coronavirus proteins, thanks to its AlphaFold artificial intelligence system **[78]**.

5.2.2.3. Discovery of bioactive molecules

BenevolentAI is a British start-up that exploits the capabilities of AI to search for and discover drugs based on their chemical properties **[79]**. It uses a vast medical database structured as a knowledge graph containing multiple links extracted from the scientific literature using ML techniques. More specifically, it uses Graphical Convolutional Neural Networks (GCNN) to extract relevant information from scientific texts and create this knowledge graph **[80]**. Her researchers have used this tool to scrutinise approved drugs, targeting those that could hinder the infection, such as inhibitors of the AAK1 enzyme, known regulators of endocytosis. With this in mind, they have highlighted a potential treatment for COVID-19. The results of their research, using the AI-based knowledge graph, identified 378 AAK1 inhibitors, 47 of which have been approved for medical use, and 6 of which inhibit AAK1 with high affinity. These include several drugs used in oncology, such as Sunitinib and Erlotinib, which have been shown to be effective in preventing viral infection of cells. However, these compounds have serious side effects, and their data suggest that high doses are required to inhibit AAK1 effectively. On the other hand, among the 6 drugs that bind with high affinity to AAK1, we find Baricitinib, a janus kinase inhibitor, which also binds to another regulator of endocytosis. Given that the plasma concentration of Baricitinib is sufficient to inhibit AAK1 with therapeutic doses of 2 mg or 4 mg, the authors suggested that it could be tested on patients with COVID-19 in order to reduce viral entry and inflammation **[79]**.Similarly, the team of Song et al. published a meta-analysis which demonstrated that Baricitinib reduced mortality and the need for mechanical ventilation in patients with severe COVID-19, confirming the suggestions of the BenevolentAI company **[81]** .

5.2.2.4. Tracking variants

During the COVID-19 health crisis, InstaDeep, a start-up founded in Tunisia and later acquired by the German giant BioNTech, developed an mRNA vaccine against Covid-19. As a result of this collaboration, an AI innovation laboratory has been set up to design a tool for assessing Sars-Cov-2 variants, the EWS (Early Warning System). automated early detection of high-risk variants of the virus **[82]**.During the pandemic, a number of SARS-Cov-2 variants were discovered, and some even posed an increased risk, due to acquired mutations favouring better evasion of antibody neutralisation or increased transmissibility.

To achieve this, the researchers aimed to combine AI with immunology. They proposed a new in silico approach that combines in-depth structural modelling of the interaction between the receptor binding domain of the Spike protein and the host cell receptor, making it possible to assess the impact of the viral variant on immune response evasion, and predictive modelling based on NLP-type AI techniques to analyse and interpret S protein sequences, in order to accurately classify SARS-CoV-2 variants **[82]**. These two parameters were validated in vitro and then merged to create EWS, which is capable of assessing new variants within minutes and monitoring variant lines in near-real time. The training data for the AI model were S protein sequences that were collected from GISAID, a global database that collects and shares genomic data on influenza and other respiratory viruses, including SARS-CoV-2 **[83]**. Several data cleaning procedures have been carried out, including the deletion of sequences that do not meet the basic biological hypotheses, sequences with more than ten continuous amino acid mutations, and sequences whose submission date was more than two months after its collection date **[82]**. In this way, the EWS assesses both the immune evasion potential and the transmission capacity of the virus, providing a

combined score for assessing the risk associated with a specific variant. This approach is highly predictive of epidemiological risk, because it integrates the two parameters. A high score indicates an increased risk of global impact of the variant. In addition, EWS allows SARS-CoV-2 variants to be classified according to their immune escape and infectivity characteristics on the basis of available data alone, without the need for subsequent data on their effects.
According to the published results, during the period from September 2020 to November 2021, a weekly analysis was carried out, identifying 90% of the variants listed by the WHO as "variants of interest" and "variants of concern", almost two months before these variants were officially designated by the WHO **[82]**. When the Alpha and Mu variants were detected by EWS, only 25 cases had been reported, while the WHO only issued an alert after around 1,500 cases had been recorded. The Omicron variant was rapidly categorised as a high-risk variant by the EWS within 24 hours of the publication of its genetic sequence. It stood out for its high level of immune evasion and its high infectious score among the tens of thousands of variants discovered during the health crisis **[82]**.
To further validate the EWS, the researchers applied standard machine learning techniques for comparison. Both supervised and unsupervised machine learning approaches were tested. For unsupervised learning, a technique called UMAP was used, but only 9 of the 16 variants were detected with an average delay of 8 days after designation by the WHO **[82]**. For supervised learning, a generalized linear model was explored, but only 8 of the 16 variants were detected early, with an average delay of 10 days after WHO designation **[82]**. In summary, these standard machine learning techniques do not achieve the predictive performance of EWS. In fact, this comparison highlights the superior performance of the EWS in the early detection of SARS-CoV-2 variants, thanks to its approach combining the two types of modelling structural and predictive, giving it a significant advantage over standard ML techniques.

5.2.3. Pharmacovigilance

In response to the thalidomide tragedy in the early 1960s, the WHO set up the pharmacovigilance programme to establish global monitoring of medicines **[84]**. Pharmacovigilance encompasses the science and actions related to the identification, assessment, understanding and prevention of adverse drug reactions and other related problems. On a global scale, pharmacovigilance collects a considerable mass of data every day, which represents a considerable processing challenge **[85]**. The exploitation of digital tools to analyse data from adverse reaction reporting databases offers encouraging prospects. For example, Kiryu and colleagues have developed an adverse drug reaction analysis system that uses machine learning to mine the Japanese Adverse Drug Event Report (JADER), a national database in Japan that collects adverse drug event reports **[86]**. The reports collected in JADER come from a variety of sources, including healthcare professionals, patients and drug manufacturers. Thus, this AI system was developed with the aim of identifying and analysing trends in drug side effects. Using machine learning, these scientists seek to extract meaningful information from the massive JADER data in order to better understand drug side-effect profiles, detect new associations between drugs and adverse effects, and potentially improve the safety and efficacy of drugs. The system was created using the C# programming language (Microsoft corporation) and the open source ML library Accord.Net Machine. Learning Framework" **[86]**. To set up this system, they produced a volcano-shaped plot, widely used in the field of toxicology for instant visualisation of the links between each drug and its side effects. They then integrated a clustering analysis into this plot

"In this way, they visually improved the trends in the groups of data relating to the side effects of drugs, by classifying them into clusters using machine learning. In this way, they visually enhanced the trends in groups of data relating to drug side effects, by classifying them into clusters using machine learning. According to the authors, the different results produced by machine learning are simply 'predictions' of the data provided by humans, and are not results calculated by statistical analyses highlighting causal relationships. In other words, this type of approach does not necessarily lead to results that can be quickly judged, up to and including a revision of a medicine's package leaflet. Of course, a machine learning method that has been properly validated could be considered reliable for analysing results, but it is important to recognise that it does not necessarily include a causal or meaningful interpretation **[86]**.

Consequently, whether for risk management using statistical analysis methods or machine learning methods, verification, investigation and evaluation of the results analysed must be considered indispensable elements. Furthermore, the results obtained by machine learning depend largely on the quality of the database, pre-processing and validation. It is therefore important to consider them as one of the criteria for interpreting the results. The application of AI in pharmacovigilance has also been described by Salas and colleagues **[87]**. They have highlighted the beneficial impact of machine learning on pharmacovigilance processes. The new modern electronic methods, such as online or mobile applications developed with the help of AI, bring a new dimension to pharmacovigilance. complementarity, simplification and extension to the ability to exchange and retrieve essential information on drug safety. They also help to improve therapeutic compliance and reduce the side effects associated with polypharmacy **[88]**. According to Litviova et al, reducing human involvement in the day-to-day operations of collecting, capturing, validating and analysing data reduces the likelihood of errors and improves the quality and accuracy of results **[89]**. Machine learning algorithms in pharmacovigilance systems can automatically analyse and filter adverse event data, enabling more effective monitoring and response to anomalies. Thus, information extraction using AI, machine learning and other digital technologies facilitates the assessment of emerging adverse drug reactions.

To conclude this section, we have drawn up a table summarising the examples of applications of AI tools mentioned in this manuscript (**Appendix 1**). Similarly, the various pharmaceutical and medical applications of machine learning methods are given in **Appendix 2**, taken from the publication by Vamathevan J et al **[90]**.

CONCLUSION

In this work, an in-depth analysis of recent research and developments in the field of AI applied to medicine and pharmacy was carried out. The various contributions The papers highlighted the transformative potential of AI in these sectors, highlighting significant advances in areas such as medical imaging, disease diagnosis, disease prediction, drug discovery and pharmacovigilance.

The findings of this analysis clearly demonstrated that AI offers unprecedented opportunities to improve the accuracy, efficiency and accessibility of healthcare. Applications of AI, such as deep ensemble models for the diagnosis of autism spectrum disorders, early warning systems for the detection of COVID-19 variants and drug discovery algorithms, have shown promising results and significant advances in clinical practice and pharmaceutical research. However, this analysis also highlighted the limitations associated with the use of AI in healthcare, particularly with regard to regulatory, ethical and security issues. It is imperative that these challenges are addressed, with particular attention paid to the protection of personal data, transparency of algorithms and resilience to cyber-attacks, to ensure responsible and ethical use of these technologies. Overcoming these problems and proposing constructive solutions will require a multidisciplinary approach, innovative data annotation methods and the development of more rigorous AI techniques and models. The creation of practical, usable and successfully implemented technologies will be possible by ensuring appropriate cooperation between computer scientists and healthcare providers. This collaboration, based on sound regulatory frameworks and increased transparency, would maximise the benefits of AI in healthcare while minimising the potential risks. In addition, collaboration between healthcare institutions is needed to share data and ensure its quality, as well as to verify the results analysed, which will be essential to the success of AI in clinical practice. Another suggestion to address the challenges of AI would be to provide appropriate training and education for all healthcare professionals, starting at university level, and to continue the continuous development and improvement of practitioners to ensure proper adaptation of AI in healthcare and to ensure the best patient care.

BIBLIOGRAPHICAL REFERENCES

1. World Health Organization. Global action on patient safety. Geneva: WHO; 2019

2. Ramdas N. Basic fundamentals of python programming language and the bright future. An Int Multi Quarterly Res J. 2019;8:71-6.

3. Cutting V, Stephen N. A review on using python as a preferred programming language for beginners. Int Res J Eng Technol. 2021;8:4258-63.

4. Chauviere L, Hoffbeck L, Shoaib M, Tessier F, Firat H, Satagopam V, et al. Firalink: A bioinformatics pipeline for long non-coding RNA data analysis. Noncoding RNA Res. 2023;8(4):602-4.

5. Brachet. Introduction to python : from algorithmic natural language to writing small python scripts [Online]. 2014 [Accessed 22/02/2024]. Availabl sur:https://www.xm1math.net/aly/assets/files/initiationpython.pdf

6. Lebigdata. Python : Tout savoir sur ce langage Big Data [Online]. 2024 [Accessed le 22/02/2024]. Available at: https://www.lebigdata.fr/python-langage

7. Dhruv AJ, Patel R, Doshi N. Python: The most advanced programming language for computer science applications: In: Proceedings of the international conference on culture heritage, education, sustainable tourism, and innovation technologies. Medan, Indonesia: Scitepress - Science and Technology Publications; 2020. p. 292-9.

8. Gupta R, Srivastava D, Sahu M, Tiwari S, Ambasta RK, Kumar P. Artificial intelligence to deep learning: Machine intelligence approach for drug discovery. Mol Divers. 2021;25(3):1315-60.

9. Tonyloi I. Building machine learning models [Online]. 2021 [Consulted on 22/02/2024]. Available at: https://www.researchgate.net/publication/349881320_Building_Machine_Learning_Models

10. Madhavan S. Build and test your first machine learning model using Python and scikit-learn [Online]. 2019 [Accessed 23/02/2024]. Available from: https://developer.ibm.com/tutorials/build-and-test-your-first-machine- learning-model-using-python-and-scikit-learn/

11. Zipfel J, Verworner F, Fischer M, Wieland U, Kraus M, Zschech P. Anomaly detection for industrial quality assurance: A comparative evaluation of unsupervised deep learning models. Comput Ind Eng. 2023;177:1-17.

12. Vos G, Trinh K, Sarnyai Z, Rahimi Azghadi M. Generalizable machine

learning for stress monitoring from wearable devices: A systematic literature review. Int J Med Inf. 2023;173:1-15.
13. Chen Z, Wong IH, Dai W, Lo CT, Wong TT. Lung cancer diagnosis on virtual histologically stained tissue using weakly supervised learning. Mod Pathol. 2024;37(6):1-12.
14. Hobensack M, Song J, Scharp D, Bowles KH, Topaz M. Machine learning applied to electronic health record data in home healthcare: A scoping review. Int J Med Inf. 2023;170:1-38.
15. Oh SH, Park J, Lee SJ, Kang S, Mo J. Reinforcement learning-based expanded personalized diabetes treatment recommendation using South Korean electronic health records. Expert Syst Appl. 2022;206:117932.
16. Data Science Test. Reinforcement Learning: Definition and Application [Online]. 2020 [Accessed 22/02/2024]. Available from: https://datascientest.com/reinforcement-learning

17. Armoogum S, Li X. Big data analytics and deep learning in bioinformatics with hadoop. In: Sangaiah AK, editor. Deep learning and parallel computing environment for bioengineering systems. Cambridge: Academic Press; 2019. p. 17-36.
18. Airiau S. Reinforcement learning [Online]. 2017 [Accessed 23/02/2024]. Available at: https://www.lamsade.dauphine.fr/~airiau/Teaching/M2-ISI-RL/2017/marl- 01-rl.pdf
19. LaBarre MO. Multi-agent learning [Online]. 2020 [Accessed 23/02/2024]. Available at: https://www.emse.fr/~boissier/enseignement/sma05/exposes/marcolivier.pd f
20. Thiry L. Fundamentals of deep learning [Online]. 2013 [Accessed 23/02/2024]. Available at: https://www.di.ens.fr/louis.thiry/slides_J1
21. IBM. What is a neural network? [Online]. 2023 [Accessed 23/02/2024]. Available at: https://www.ibm.com/fr-fr/topics/neural- networks
22. Chen EZ, Wang P, Chen X, Chen T, Sun S. Pyramid convolutional RNN for MRI image reconstruction. IEEE Trans Med Imaging. 2022;41(8):2033-47.
23. Baur C, Denner S, Wiestler B, Navab N, Albarqouni S. Autoencoders for unsupervised anomaly segmentation in brain MR images: A comparative study. Med Image Anal. 2021;69:1-16.
24. Rong R, Jiang S, Xu L, Xiao G, Xie Y, Liu DJ, et al. MB-GAN: Microbiome simulation via generative adversarial network. GigaScience. 2021;10(2):1- 11.
25. Mathew S, Nadeem S, Kaufman A. CLTS-GAN: Color-lighting-texture-specular reflection augmentation for colonoscopy. Med Image Comput Comput

Assist Interv. 2022;2022:519-29.

26. Pan Y, Liu J, Cai Y, Yang X, Zhang Z, Long H, et al. Fundus image classification using Inception V3 and ResNet-50 for the early diagnostics of fundus diseases. Front Physiol. 2023;14:1-9.
27. Moezzi SA, Ghaedi A, Rahmanian M, Mousavi SZ, Sami A. Application of deep learning in generating structured radiology reports: A transformer- based technique. J Digit Imaging. 2023;36(1):80-90.
28. Ljubic B, Hai AA, Stanojevic M, Diaz W, Polimac D, Pavlovski M, et al. Predicting complications of diabetes mellitus using advanced machine learning algorithms. J Am Med Inform Assoc. 2020;27(9):1343-51.
29. Jones A, Gandhi V, Mahiddine AY, Huyck C. Bridging neuroscience and robotics: Spiking neural networks in action. Sensors. 2023;23(21):1-14.
30. Fu S, Wang X, Tang J, Lan S, Tian Y. Generalized robust loss functions for machine learning. Neural Netw. 2024;171:200-14.
31. Olsen F, Schillaci C, Ibrahim M, Lipani A. Borough-level COVID-19 forecasting in London using deep learning techniques and a novel MSE-Moran's I loss function. Results Phys. 2022;35:1-13.
32. Rajendran R, Karthi A. Heart disease prediction using entropy based feature engineering and ensembling of machine learning classifiers. Expert Syst Appl. 2022;207:117882.
33. Fürst F. History of Artificial Intelligence [Online]. 2014 [Accessed 23/04/2024]. Available at: https://home.mis.u-picardie.fr/~furst/docs/3-Naissance_IA.pdf
34. Chen G, Huang B, Chen X, Ge L, Radenkovic M, Ma Y. Deep blue AI: A new bridge from data to knowledge for the ocean science. Deep Sea Res Part Oceanogr Res Pap. 2022;190:103886.
35. Wang S. Factors related to user perceptions of artificial intelligence (AI)-based content moderation on social media. Comput Hum Behav. 2023;149:107971.

36. Manaouil C, Chamot S, Petit P. Le médecin confronté à l'AI (Intelligence artificielle): Ethics and responsibility. Med Droit. 2024 [In press]. https://doi.org/10.1016/j.meddro.2024.02.001
37. Do S, Song KD, Chung JW. Basics of deep learning: A radiologist's guide to understanding published radiology articles on deep learning. Korean J Radiol. 2019;21(1):33-41.
38. Sharma S. Benefits or concerns of AI: A multistakeholder responsibility. Futures. 2024;157:1-10.

39. Papadimitriou E, Schneider C, Aguinaga Tello J, Damen W, Lomba Vrouenraets M, ten Broeke A. Transport safety and human factors in the era of automation: What can transport modes learn from each other? Accid Anal Prev. 2020;144:1-16.
40. Ahmed I, Kajol MA, Hasan U, Datta PP. ChatGPT vs. Bard: A comparative study [OnlineOnline]. 2023 [Consult the 22/02/2024]. Available at: https://www.researchgate.net/publication/371799069_ChatGPT_vs_Bard_ A_Comparative_Study
41. Botco. GenAI Chatbots inmarketing [Online]. 2024 [Accessed 13/04/2024]. Available sur: https://botco.ai/wp- content/uploads/Botco.ai_The-State-of-GenAI-Chatbots-in-Marketing_- Digital-Report_V4.pdf
42. Pai KC, Kuo BC, Liao CH, Liu YM. An application of Chinese dialogue-based intelligent tutoring system in remedial instruction for mathematics learning. Educ Psychol. 2021;41(2):137-52.
43. Hwang GJ, Sung HY, Chang SC, Huang XC. A fuzzy expert system-based adaptive learning approach to improving students' learning performances by considering affective and cognitive factors. Comput Educ Artif Intell. 2020;1:1-15.

44. Myszczynska MA, Ojamies PN, Lacoste AM, Neil D, Saffari A, Mead R, et al. Applications of machine learning to diagnosis and treatment of neurodegenerative diseases. Nat Rev Neurol. 2020;16(8):440-56.
45. Landau MS, Pantanowitz L. Artificial intelligence in cytopathology: A review of the literature and overview of commercial landscape. J Am Soc Cytopathol. 2019;8(4):230-41.
46. Quazi S. Artificial intelligence and machine learning in precision and genomic medicine. Med Oncol. 2022;39(8):1-18.
47. Johnson KB, Wei WQ, Weeraratne D, Frisse ME, Misulis K, Rhee K, et al. Precision medicine, AI, and the future of personalized health care. Clin Transl Sci. 2021;14(1):86-93.
48. Blasiak A, Truong A, Tan WJ, Kumar KS, Tan SB, Teo CB, et al. Precise curate.AI: A prospective feasibility trial to dynamically modulate personalized chemotherapy dose with artificial intelligence. J Clin Oncol. 2022;40(16):1574.
49. Gerke S, Minssen T, Cohen G. Ethical and legal challenges of artificial intelligence-driven healthcare. In: Bohr A, Memarzadeh K, editors. Artificial intelligence in healthcare. Cambridge: Academic Press; 2020. p. 295-336.
50. Yuan B, Li J. The policy effect of the general data protection regulation (GDPR) on the digital public health sector in the European Union: An empirical investigation. Int J Environ Res Public Health. 2019;16(6):1-15.

51. Hazarika I. Artificial intelligence: Opportunities and implications for the health workforce. Int Health. 2020;12(4):241-5.
52. Ahsan MM, Luna SA, Siddique Z. Machine-learning-based disease diagnosis: A comprehensive review. Healthcare. 2022;10(3):1-30.

53. Xu H, Shuttleworth KM. Medical artificial intelligence and the black box problem: A view based on the ethical principle of "do no harm". Intell Med. 2024;4(1):52-7.
54. Mittermaier M, Raza MM, Kvedar JC. Bias in AI-based models for medical applications: Challenges and mitigation strategies. Npj Digit Med. 2023;6(1):1-3.
55. Chin MH, Afsar-Manesh N, Bierman AS, Chang C, Colón-Rodríguez CJ, Dullabh P, et al. Guiding principles to address the impact of algorithm bias on racial and ethnic disparities in health and health care. JAMA Netw Open. 2023;6(12):1-13.
56. Buslón N, Cortés A, Catuara-Solarz S, Cirillo D, Rementeria MJ. Raising awareness of sex and gender bias in artificial intelligence and health. Front Glob Womens Health. 2023;4:1-8.
57. Alowais SA, Alghamdi SS, Alsuhebany N, Alqahtani T, Alshaya AI, Almohareb SN, et al. Revolutionizing healthcare: The role of artificial intelligence in clinical practice. BMC Med Educ. 2023;23(1):1-15.
58. World Health Organization. WHO outlines considerations for regulation of artificial intelligence for health. Geneva: WHO; 2023.
59. Tenajas R, Miraut D, Illana CI, Alonso-Gonzalez R, Arias-Valcayo F, Herraiz JL. Recent advances in artificial intelligence-assisted ultrasound scanning. Appl Sci. 2023;13(6):1-17.
60. Fiorentino MC, Villani FP, Di Cosmo M, Frontoni E, Moccia S. A review on deep-learning algorithms for fetal ultrasound-image analysis. Med Image Anal. 2023;83:1-31.
61. Tayebi Arasteh S, Misera L, Kather JN, Truhn D, Nebelung S. Enhancing diagnostic deep learning via self-supervised pretraining on large-scale, unlabeled non-medical images. Eur Radiol Exp. 2024;8(1):1-17.

62. Kim JH, Hong J, Choi H, Kang HG, Yoon S, Hwang JY, et al. Development of deep ensembles to screen for autism and symptom severity using retinal photographs. JAMA Netw Open. 2023;6(12):1-12.
63. Weisenburger RL, Mullarkey MC, Labrada J, Labrousse D, Yang MY, MacPherson AH, et al. Conversational assessment using artificial intelligence is as clinically useful as depression scales and preferred by users. J Affect Disord.

2024;351:489-98.
64. Kanda F, Oishi K, Sekiguchi K, Kuga A, Kobessho H, Shirafuji T, et al. Characteristics of depression in Parkinson's disease: Evaluating with Zung's Self-Rating depression scale. Parkinson Relat Disord. 2008;14(1):19-23.
65. Lim JI, Regillo CD, Sadda SR, Ipp E, Bhaskaranand M, Ramachandra C, et al. Artificial intelligence detection of diabetic retinopathy: Subgroup comparison of the EyeArt system with ophthalmologists' dilated examinations. Ophthalmol Sci. 2023;3(1):1-8.
66. Placido D, Yuan B, Hjaltelin JX, Zheng C, Haue AD, Chmura PJ, et al. A deep learning algorithm to predict risk of pancreatic cancer from disease trajectories. Nat Med. 2023;29(5):1113-22.
67. Gao Y, Cai GY, Fang W, Li HY, Wang SY, Chen L, et al. Machine learning based early warning system enables accurate mortality risk prediction for COVID-19. Nat Commun. 2020;11(1):1-10.
68. Li QY, An ZY, Pan ZH, Wang ZZ, Wang YR, Zhang XG, et al. Severe/critical COVID-19 early warning system based on machine learning algorithms using novel imaging scores. World J Clin Cases. 2023;11(12):2716-28.
69. Jin S, Liu G, Bai Q. Deep learning in COVID-19 diagnosis, prognosis and treatment selection. Mathematics. 2023;11(6):1-16.

70. Stokes JM, Yang K, Swanson K, Jin W, Cubillos-Ruiz A, Donghia NM, et al. A deep learning approach to antibiotic discovery. Cell. 2020;180(4):688- 702.
71. Junaid M, Thirapanmethee K, Khuntayaporn P, Chomnawang MT. CRISPR-based gene editing in acinetobacter baumannii to combat antimicrobial resistance. Pharmaceuticals. 2023;16(7):1-32.
72. Mellouli A, Maamar B, Bouzakoura F, Messadi AA, Thabet L. Colonisation and infection with acinetobacter baumannii in a burns resuscitation unit in Tunisia. Ann Burns Fire Disasters. 2021;34(3):218-25.
73. Liu G, Catacutan DB, Rathod K, Swanson K, Jin W, Mohammed JC, et al. Deep learning-guided discovery of an antibiotic targeting acinetobacter baumannii. Nat Chem Biol. 2023;19(11):1342-50.
74. Parasher A. COVID-19: Current understanding of its pathophysiology, clinical presentation and treatment. Postgrad Med J. 2021;97:312-20.
75. Kricka LJ, Polevikov S, Park JY, Fortina P, Bernardini S, Satchkov D, et al. Artificial intelligence-powered search tools and resources in the fight against COVID-19. EJIFCC. 2020;31(2):106-16.
76. Jin Q, Leaman R, Lu Z. PubMed and beyond: Biomedical literature search in the age of artificial intelligence. EBioMedicine. 2024;100:1-12.

77. Huang L, Zhang H, Deng D, Zhao K, Liu K, Hendrix DA, et al. LinearFold: Linear-time approximate RNA folding by 5'-to-3' dynamic programming and beam search. Bioinformatics. 2019;35(14):295-304.
78. Thornton JM, Laskowski RA, Borkakoti N. AlphaFold heralds a data-driven revolution in biology and medicine. Nat Med. 2021;27(10):1666-9.
79. Richardson P, Griffin I, Tucker C, Smith D, Oechsle O, Phelan A, et al. Baricitinib as potential treatment for 2019-nCoV acute respiratory disease. Lancet. 2020;395:30-1.

80. Santana MV, Silva FP. Artificial intelligence methods to repurpose and discover new drugs to fight the Coronavirus disease-2019 pandemic. In: Panda S, Kumari L, Badwaik HR, Shanmugarajan D, editors. Computational approaches for novel therapeutic and diagnostic designing to mitigate SARS-CoV-2 Infection. Cambridge: Academic Press; 2022. p.537- 57.
81. Song W, Sun S, Feng Y, Liu L, Gao T, Xian S, et al. Efficacy and safety of baricitinib in patients with severe COVID-19: A systematic review and meta-analysis. Medicine. 2023;102(48):1-7.
82. Beguir K, Skwark MJ, Fu Y, Pierrot T, Carranza NL, Laterre A, et al. Early computational detection of potential high-risk SARS-CoV-2 variants. Comput Biol Med. 2023;155:1-9.
83. Khare S, Gurry C, Freitas L, Schultz MB, Bach G, Diallo A, et al. GISAID's role in pandemic response. China CDC Wkly. 2021;3(49):1049-51.

84. Gouraud A. La pharmacovigilance, principes et fonctionnement. Sages-Femmes. 2024;23(2):40-3.
85. Murali K, Kaur S, Prakash A, Medhi B. Artificial intelligence in pharmacovigilance: Practical utility. Indian J Pharmacol. 2019;51(6):373-6.
86. Kiryu Y. Potential for big data analysis using AI in the field of clinical pharmacy. Yakugaku Zasshi. 2021;141(2):179-85.
87. Salas M, Petracek J, Yalamanchili P, Aimer O, Kasthuril D, Dhingra S, et al. The use of artificial intelligence in pharmacovigilance: A systematic review of the literature. Pharm Med. 2022;36(5):295-306.
88. Akyon SH, Akyon FC, Yılmaz TE. Artificial intelligence-supported web application design and development for reducing polypharmacy side effects and supporting rational drug use in geriatric patients. Front Med. 2023;10:1- 16.

89. Litvinova O, Yeung AW, Hammerle FP, Mickael ME, Matin M, Kletecka-Pulker M, et al. Digital technology applications in the management of adverse drug reactions: Bibliometric analysis. Pharmaceuticals. 2024;17(3):1-17.

90. Vamathevan J, Clark D, Czodrowski P, Dunham I, Ferran E, Lee G, et al. Applications of machine learning in drug discovery and development. Nat Rev Drug Discov. 2019;18(6):463-77.

APPENDICES

Appendix 1: Summary of examples of applications of AI tools mentioned in this manuscript.

Domain application	Type of application	AI tool	Publication, date
Medical	Pelvic ultrasound	analysisLearning by reinforcement reinforcement learning (MARL)	[60], 2023
	Thoracic ultrasound analysisSelf-supervised	learning SSL	(61), 2024
	Autism diagnosis	Deep ensemble models with ResNeXt-50(32x4d) deep convolutional neural networks	(62), 2023
	Diagnosis of depression Diagnosis of retinopathy	: Multimodal artificial intelligence (AI) platform EyeArt: *AI* technology for autonomous detection of diabetic retinopathy	(63), 2024 (65), 2023
	Prediction of	pancreatic cancerML predictive models	(66), 2023
	Prediction of mortality risk in patients with Covid	MRPMC	(67), 2020
Pharmaceuticals	Development of antibiotics (Halicin and Abaucina)	Neural message passing network	(70), 2020 (73), 2023
	Predicting the structure of viral RNA molecules	Linearfold	(77), 2019
	Protein structure prediction	AlphaFold	(78), 2021
	Intelligent search for scientific publications AI-based visualisation of associations between concepts in the CORD-19 database	WellAI SciSight	(75), 2020 (76), 2020
	Identifying a treatment for created	COVID-19Benevolent AI: Knowledge graph by RNCG	(79), 2020
	Rapid detection of high-risk variants of the Sars Cov 2 virus	EWS: automated early warning system	(82), 2023
	Pharmacovigilance	Unsupervised *clustering* learning k-means with a Gaussian mixture model	(86), 2021

Appendix 2: Different pharmaceutical and medical applications of machine learning methods.

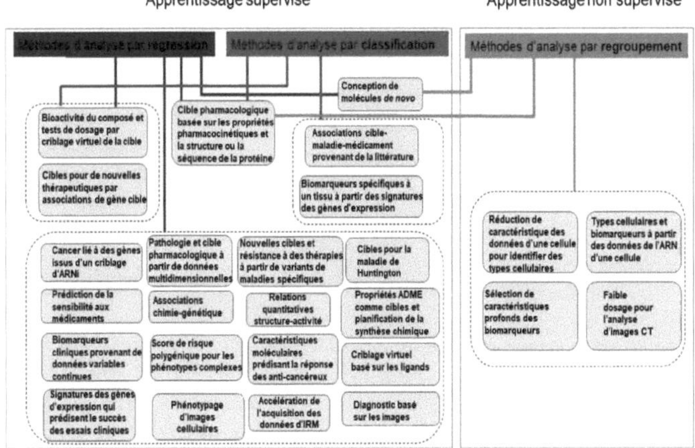

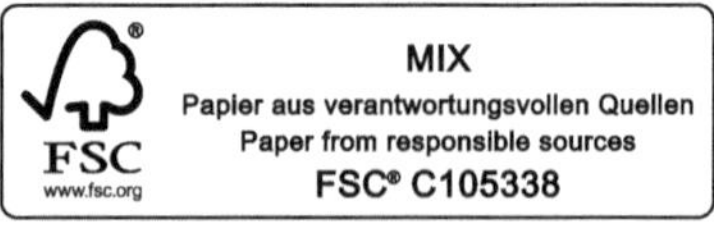

Printed by Books on Demand GmbH, Norderstedt / Germany